ICU Demystified: What Everyone Should Know

OrangeBooks Publication

1st Floor, Rajhans Arcade, Mall Road, Kohka, Bhilai, Chhattisgarh 490020

Website: **www.orangebooks.in**

First Edition, 2025

ISBN: 978-93-6554-474-9

Price: Rs. 399.00

Printed in India

ICU DEMYSTIFIED

WHAT EVERYONE SHOULD KNOW

THE BOOK YOU HOPE YOU'LL NEVER NEED - BUT MUST HAVE!

DR. CHANDRESHKUMAR SUDANI

OrangeBooks Publication
www.orangebooks.in

Acknowledgements

This book is the result of not only years of clinical experience, but also the unwavering encouragement, guidance, and love I have received from those around me. I owe deep gratitude to each of you for walking alongside me.

To my parents—your values, and unconditional love have laid the foundation for all that I do.

To my wife, **Dr.Varsha**, a gifted physician and constant source of wisdom—thank you for being my companion, and my daily inspiration.

To my family members and loved ones—your encouragement and support have always lifted me higher.

To my esteemed teachers, **Dr. Manimala Rao**, **Dr. Srinivas Samavedam, Dr. Ganshyam Jagathkar** and **Dr. Pradeep Reddy** —your mentorship and dedication continue to inspire my work in critical care.

To **Dr. M S S Mukharjee**— your experience and excellence continue to influence my communication approach to patients and their families.

To my friends in critical care medicine, **Dr. Nandhakishore**, **Dr. Mithilesh**, **Dr. Qadeer** and **Dr. Naresh**—your insights, and laughter have been my invaluable companions.

To all friends not individually named—please accept my heartfelt thanks for your invaluable support.

Dr.Chandreshkumar Sudani

(MBBS, DNB, IDCCM, PGDHHM)

Senior Critical Care Specialist

Introduction

Health is one of the most important aspects of life. Many of us have experienced the distress of having a loved one admitted to the ICU due to a serious health condition. While the patient receives care, relatives wait outside the ICU, filled with uncertainty and anxiety. Even though doctors provide regular updates, understanding complex medical terms can be challenging for individuals without any medical knowledge.

Sometimes, relatives seek explanations from their family physician or request a second opinion. However, not everyone has easy access to another doctor. Relatives are better able to understand complex health situations when they are explained in simple language.

Due to time constraints, doctors cannot answer every question asked by the relatives. Therefore, it is essential for relatives to focus on the most relevant questions related to the patient's condition. They should know the difference between general questions and specific questions. Let's understand this with example:

Patient X is admitted to the ICU with fever, cough, and breathlessness. After two days without improvement, doctors call the relatives for an update. Relatives may ask many questions, but they often include general questions such as:

- "Why can't you treat my loved one in the general ward?"
- "Why is oxygen support being used?"
- "What are the visiting hours?"
- "Can I bring other relatives to see the patient?"
- "Can I stay with the patient all day?"
- "How and how often will I get updates on my loved one's condition?"

While valid, these questions may not be specific to the patient. Instead, relatives should ask:

- "What is the final diagnosis?"
- "What treatments are being given or planned?"
- "How much oxygen support is needed today?"
- "What abnormalities were found in the blood reports?"
- "What are the next options for oxygen therapy?"
- "Is the patient showing any improvement compared to yesterday?"
- "What is the prognosis? (prognosis means chances of recovery or outcomes)

While waiting in the hospital, relatives often read newspapers or books. If they use this time to learn about the ICU and common diseases treated there, they will better understand the patient's condition and the medical discussions during counselling sessions. Reading articles, booklets, or materials written in simple language can make this knowledge more accessible. When presented in a question-and-answer format, the information becomes even easier to understand, as it reflects common doubts and concerns.

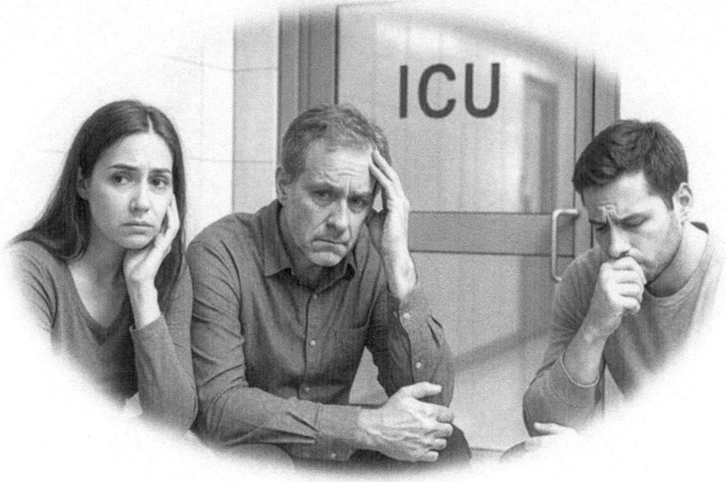

The Intensive Care Unit (ICU) is a vital area within the hospital, where critically ill patients receive constant and specialized medical care. For individuals who have never encountered this environment, stepping into the ICU for the first time can be an overwhelming experience—marked by feelings of anxiety, fear, and uncertainty. Not only patients but their families often feel apprehensive upon seeing the array of medical equipment and severely ill individuals around them.

This reaction is largely driven by unfamiliarity. A lack of basic knowledge about common medical terminology, procedures, and equipment can magnify distress. Conversely, a little awareness can transform that fear into understanding and calm. Consider this simple illustration: Patient X is admitted to the ICU for the first time due to sudden breathlessness. He and his family are visibly anxious, unsure of what lies ahead. Patient Y, admitted for the same condition but with prior ICU experience, enters the unit with relative ease. His familiarity with the environment, treatment modalities, and equipment gives him and his family a sense of reassurance.

This example reflects an important truth: patients and their families benefit greatly from having basic medical knowledge about ICU care. Understanding the physical setup of the ICU, the purpose of various devices, and how they support patient recovery can ease anxiety, empower communication with care providers, and foster comfort during ICU stay.

Contents

Chapter - 7

Chapter - 8

Chapter - 1

What is the ICU and Why is My Loved One Here?

Q1.1: What does "ICU" stand for?

ICU stands for Intensive Care Unit. It is a highly monitored area in the hospital where people with serious illnesses or injuries are admitted for close observation and advanced treatment. Most ICUs are managed by the Department of Critical Care Medicine.

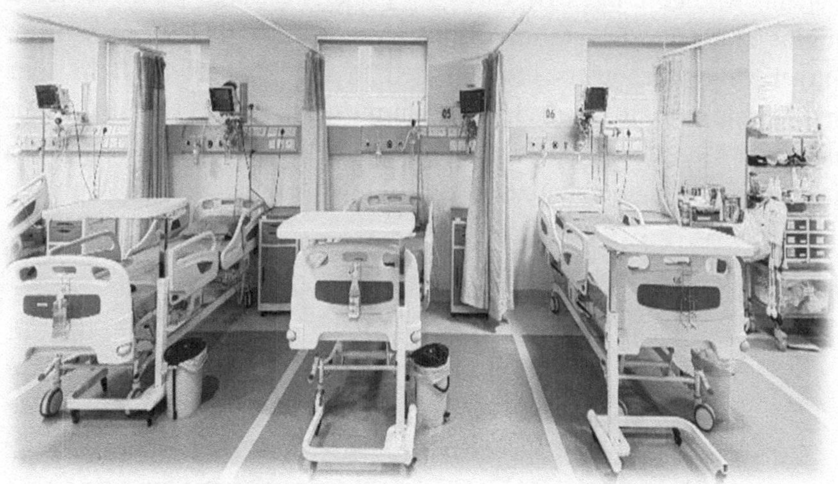

Unlike general hospital wards, the ICU is equipped with advanced monitoring equipment, specialized medical personnel, and a higher nurse-to-patient ratio. The ICU is designed to handle complex medical problems that require a higher level of care, which is difficult to provide in other areas of the hospital.

Q1.2: Why are there many different types of ICUs in a multi-specialty hospital?

There are two main types of ICUs in most hospitals:

1) Medical ICU and 2) Surgical ICU. However, many multi-specialty hospitals have specialized ICUs, which may include:

- MICU (Medical ICU)
- SICU (Surgical ICU)
- NICU (Neonatal ICU)
- PICU (Paediatric ICU)
- ICCU (Intensive Coronary Care Unit)
- RICU (Respiratory ICU)
- CTICU (Cardiothoracic ICU)

Patients who need intensive care before and after surgery may be treated in the Surgical ICU (after major surgeries) or CTICU (after heart surgeries), while others are admitted to the Medical ICU. In some multidisciplinary ICUs, medical and surgical patients are kept in the same unit with dedicated area allotment. Post-surgical care is usually provided in separate ICUs to minimize the risk of infections.

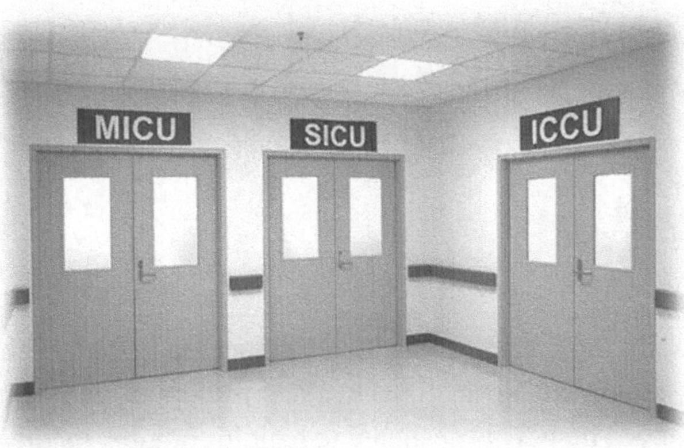

If the hospital also treats children, there may be a separate ICU for new-born babies known as the Neonatal ICU. Doctors and staff trained in specific specialties can provide better care to patients admitted to the respective ICU based on their illness.

Q1.3: Why do some patients need the ICU instead of a regular ward in hospital?

Certain clinical conditions require continuous monitoring of vital signs. These vital signs include blood pressure, heart rate, respiratory rate, oxygen saturation level, and temperature.

If patients arrive at the emergency room with abnormal vital signs, they will definitely need to stay in the ICU until they are stabilized or recovered. However, sometimes a patient may appear stable but has a medical condition that could suddenly affect the vitals. Such patients also require ICU admission even if initial vitals are normal. Some patients in the ICU may be critically ill, while others may be quite stable.

In addition to abnormal vitals, there are other reasons for ICU admission. These may include blood transfusions, chemotherapy, minor procedures, bleeding disorders, low platelet counts requiring platelet transfusions, etc.

ICU patients often need life-support treatments such as breathing assistance, medication to support heart function, or continuous monitoring that cannot be provided in rooms or general wards.

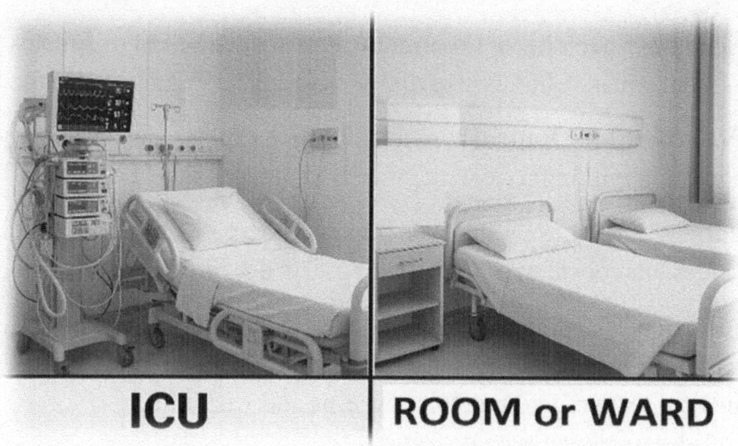

Q1.4: How is the decision made to admit someone to the ICU?

The decision to admit a patient to the ICU is made by a physician or a specialist based on a careful evaluation of the patient's medical condition and needs.

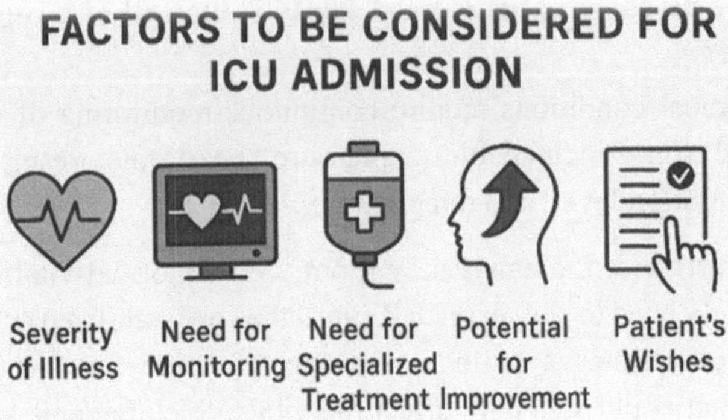

Several factors are considered, including:

- **Severity of Illness:** Patients with life-threatening conditions that require intensive medical management are typically admitted to the ICU.
- **Need for Monitoring:** Continuous monitoring of vital signs and other parameters may require ICU admission. Patient's vitals might be absolutely stable but if continuous monitoring is required, patient has to be in the ICU even with stable vitals.
- **Need for Specialized Treatment:** Patients who need treatments such as mechanical ventilation or dialysis are generally admitted to the ICU.
- **Potential for Improvement:** The possibility that the patient's condition will improve with intensive care is also a key factor.
- **Patient's Wishes:** Whenever possible, the patient's preferences and values are considered when making ICU decisions.

The decision to admit someone to the ICU can be challenging. It's important for patients and families to maintain open communication with the medical team regarding their concerns and wishes.

Chapter - 2

Understanding the ICU Environment

Q2.1: What does the ICU environment look and sound like?

The ICU environment can be very active and sometimes overwhelming. Here are some common sights and sounds:

- **Bright Lights:** ICUs are usually brightly lit to allow constant observation of patients.
- **Alarms:** Monitoring equipment may sound different alarms. These can seem distressing, but they are often routine and do not always mean something serious.
- **Beeping Sounds:** The beeping of monitors and medical equipment is commonly heard in the ICU.
- **Conversations:** The medical team is regularly communicating about patient care.
- **Medical Equipment:** The ICU contains various devices, including ventilators, monitors, and infusion pumps.

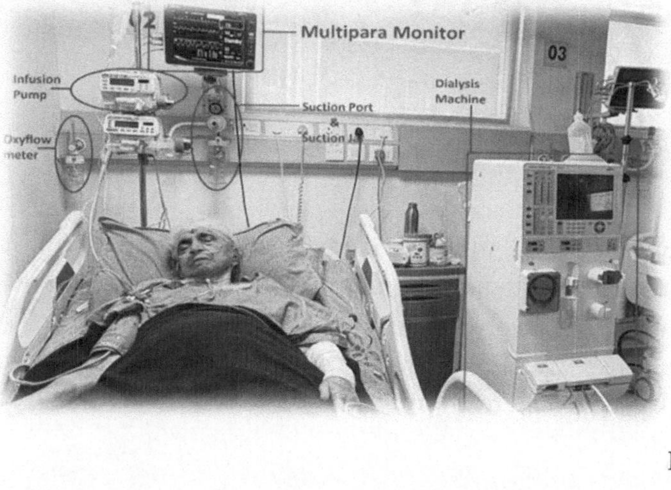

It's important to understand that the ICU environment is designed to offer the best care for critically ill patients. Although it may feel intense, the medical team is committed to creating a safe and supportive space for patients and their loved ones.

Q2.2: Which specialist doctors are involved in a patient's care in the ICU?

In most hospitals, ICUs are managed by critical care specialists. These doctors are called **intensivists**, and they care for seriously ill patients needing intensive treatment. Intensivists are trained to handle emergencies and use different life-support systems.

Some ICUs may also be managed by anaesthesiologists, emergency physicians, pulmonologists, or general physicians with experience in treating complex critical cases.

Many ICU patients may have problems affecting multiple organs, and specialists from various fields may be consulted depending on the patient's condition.

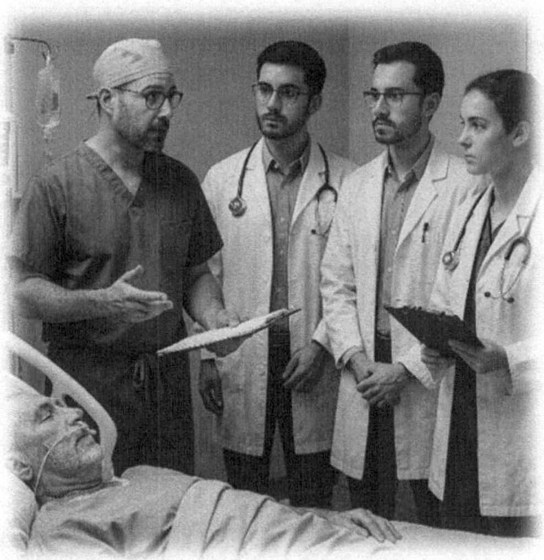

ICU care requires a **multidisciplinary approach**, where all specialist doctors collaborate to help the patient recover. If a patient needs surgery, a surgeon will be involved, and the patient may return to the ICU for post-surgery care—where physicians and surgeons continue to monitor and treat the patient until recovery.

Relatives typically receive updates from one of these doctors. It is not necessary for only a specific specialist to communicate with family members. Any doctor from the treating team may provide updates during counselling sessions.

Q2.3: Who are the key team members in the ICU?

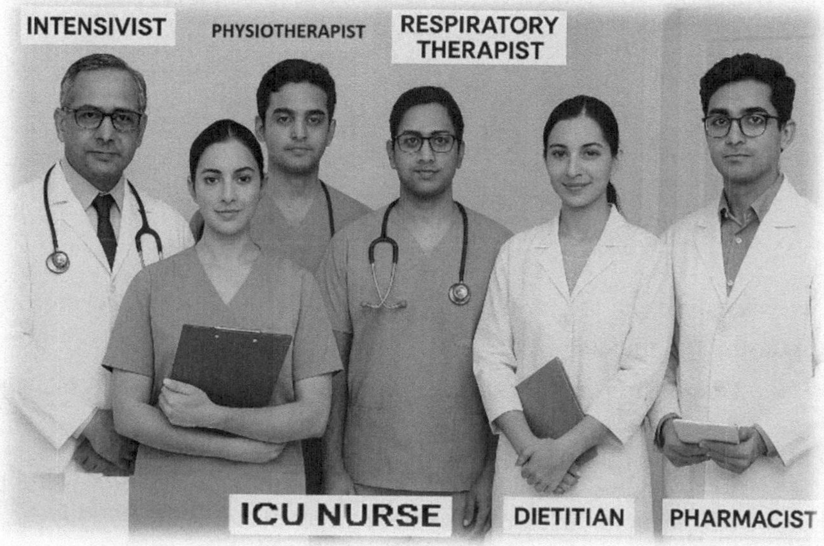

- **Intensivists:** Specialist doctors who lead patient care.
- **ICU Nurses:** Constant caregivers trained in critical care.
- **Respiratory Therapists:** Experts in managing breathing equipment.
- **Physiotherapists:** Professionals who assist with physical recovery.
- **Dietitians & Pharmacists:** Ensure proper nutrition and correct medications.

Q2.4: What is the role of the Intensivist?

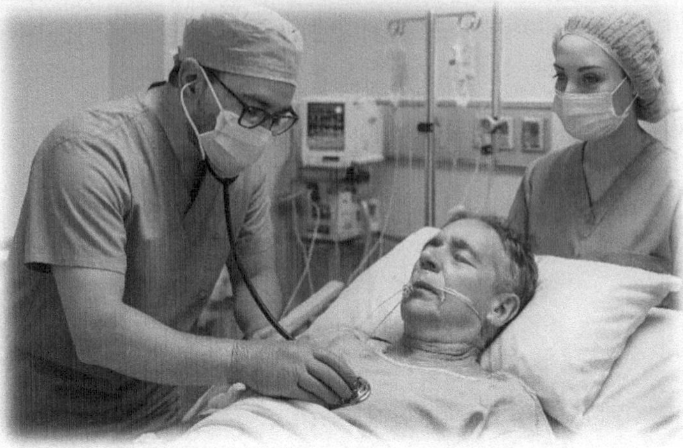

The intensivist is the primary leader of the ICU team. Their key responsibilities include:

- **Diagnosing and Treating Illnesses:** They identify and manage the conditions that led to ICU admission.
- **Creating and Managing Treatment Plans:** They work with the ICU team to develop personalized care plans.
- **Monitoring Recovery:** They track each patient's progress and adjust treatments as needed.
- **Performing Procedures:** Intensivists carry out procedures like:
    - Inserting **central lines** near the neck or collarbone to give multiple medicines at once
    - Placing **arterial lines** near the wrist or groin to monitor blood pressure continuously
    - Starting **invasive ventilation support** when required
- **Communicating with Families:** They explain the patient's condition, treatments, and expected progress.
- **Coordinating with Other Doctors:** They work closely with other specialists to ensure patients receive comprehensive care.

Q2.5: What is the role of the ICU nurses?

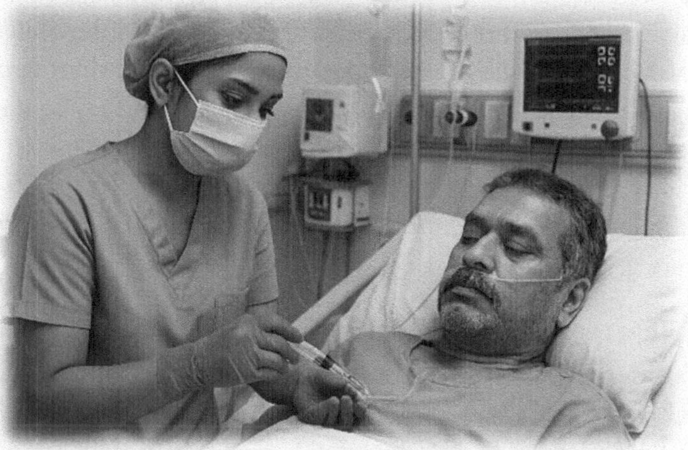

ICU nurses are the frontline caregivers in the ICU. Their key duties include:

- **Monitoring Vital Signs:** They check heart rate, blood pressure, oxygen level, and breathing regularly.
- **Giving Medications:** Nurses administer medicines as prescribed by doctors.
- **Performing Procedures:** They insert IV (intravenous) lines, draw blood, and change wound dressings.
- **Offering Personal Care:** Nurses help with bathing, feeding, and changing linens.
- **Providing Emotional Support:** They comfort both patients and their families.
- **Noticing and Responding to Changes:** ICU nurses are trained to quickly recognize any changes in condition and act promptly.
- **Documenting Care:** Nurses carefully record every aspect of care—vitals, medications, and treatments—ensuring the team has accurate information for decision-making.

Q2.6: How often do nurses and doctors check on patients?

ICU patients are never left unattended. Nurses provide round-the-clock care, and doctors visit regularly—often several times a day. Intensivists are always present in the ICU and monitor patients' vital signs frequently. Although they may be attending to the sickest patients, they continuously observe and respond to the needs of all ICU patients. If intensivist is busy in providing emergency treatment to another patient at different area of the hospital, junior doctor might be monitoring the ICU patients while ICU nurses are giving treatment to patients.

Q2.7: What are the different devices commonly seen in the ICU?

1. **Multipara Monitor:** This is a small screen located at the head of the ICU bed, showing 5 to 7 vital parameters (ECG, heart rate, Oxygen level, blood pressure, breathing rate)

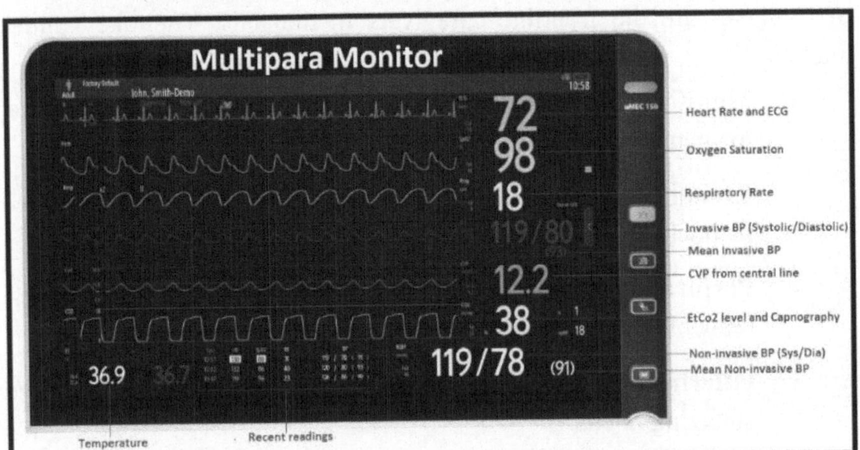

- **ECG (Electrocardiogram):** Tracks the electrical activity of the heart using chest electrodes.
- **HR (Heart Rate):** Shows the number of heart beats per minute. A normal range is 60–100 per minute.
- **SpO_2 (Peripheral Oxygen Saturation):** Indicates the percentage of oxygen in the body using a pulse oximeter attached to a finger. Normal is 95% or above.
- **PR (Pulse Rate):** Also measured by the pulse oximeter; always matches the heart rate.

- **BP (Blood Pressure):** Measured with a BP cuff on the arm or leg, or continuously via an arterial catheter in very sick patients. Readings from arterial catheters usually appear in red on the monitor.
- **Temperature:** Continuously monitored using a probe placed in the nose. (only required for certain clinical conditions)
- **$EtCO_2$ (End-Tidal Carbon Dioxide):** Measures the level of carbon dioxide in exhaled breath, typically in ventilated patients.

The monitor produces a beeping sound with each heartbeat to alert nurses and doctors to any sudden changes. Though the sound might be annoying, it is vital—even when patients are asleep.

2. **Infusion Pumps:** These pumps deliver precise doses of medication through a syringe fixed into the pump. They are commonly used for drugs like vasopressors (drugs to raise BP), inotropes (drugs to improve heart function), cardiac medications, blood pressure medications, antibiotics, and others.

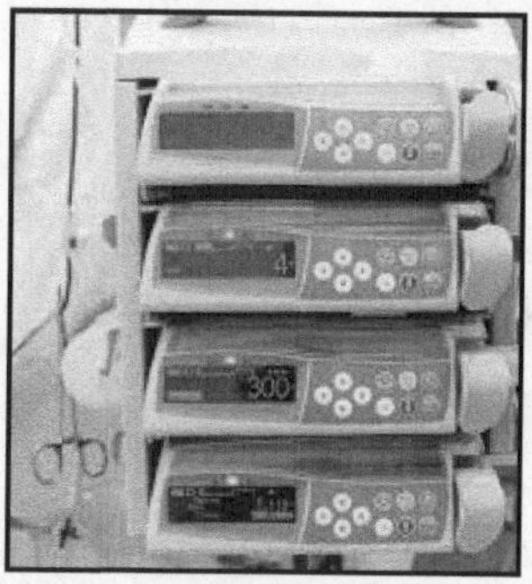

3. **Oxyflow Meter:** A wall-mounted device that delivers oxygen to the patient through a nasal cannula or mask, up to 15 litres per minute. It can also be used for nebulization therapy.

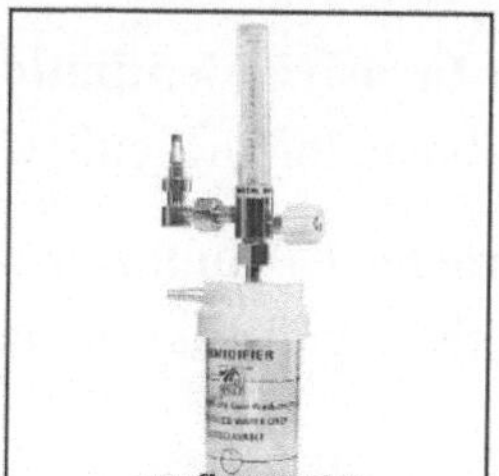

oxyflow meter

4. **Suction Jar:** A transparent jar near the head of the ICU bed that helps suction secretions from the mouth using a tube. It is used to clear blood, mucus, or other fluids.

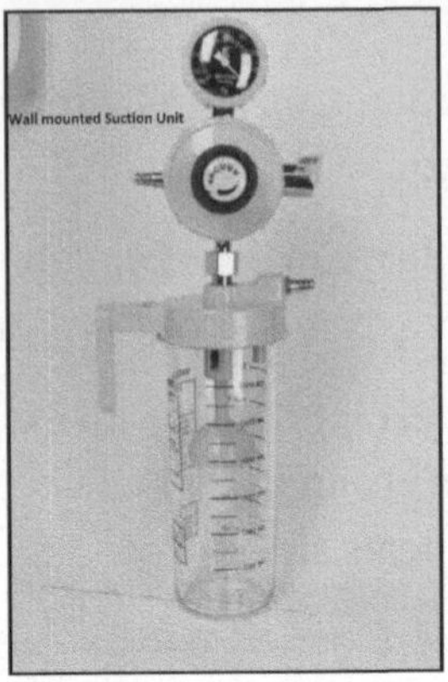

5. **Ventilator:** This machine helps or takes over breathing for patients who cannot breathe properly.

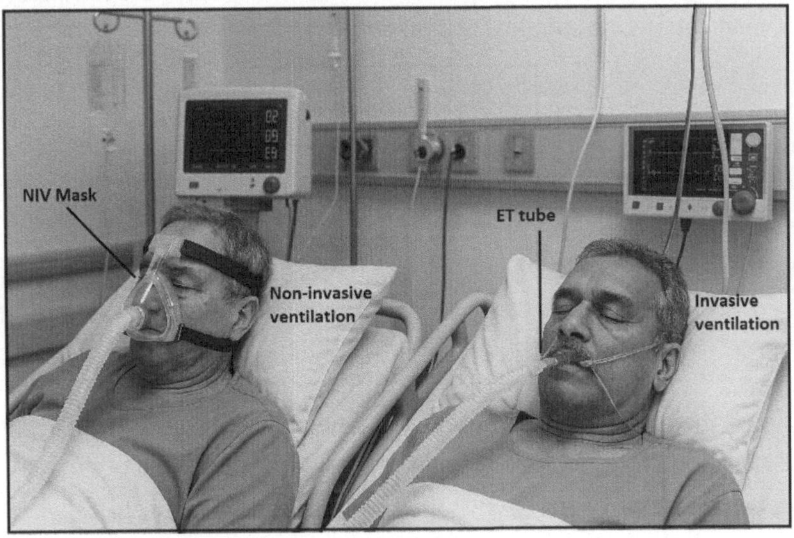

- **NIV Mask (Non-Invasive Ventilation):** Used if the patient is conscious but has breathing difficulty.
- **ET Tube (Endotracheal Tube):** A breathing tube in the windpipe for the patients with lung disease or altered conscious level.

6. **Dialysis Machine:** Different machines are used for kidney support in ICU patients.

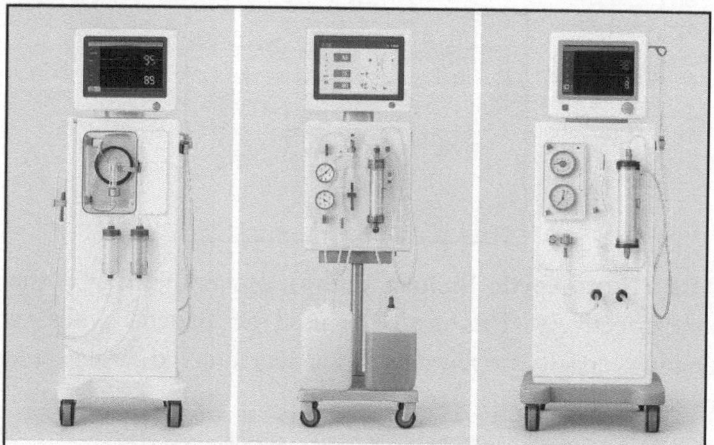

Different Types of Dialysis Machines

7. **Defibrillator:** Used to deliver a DC (Direct Current) shock in cases of life-threatening heart rhythm problems.

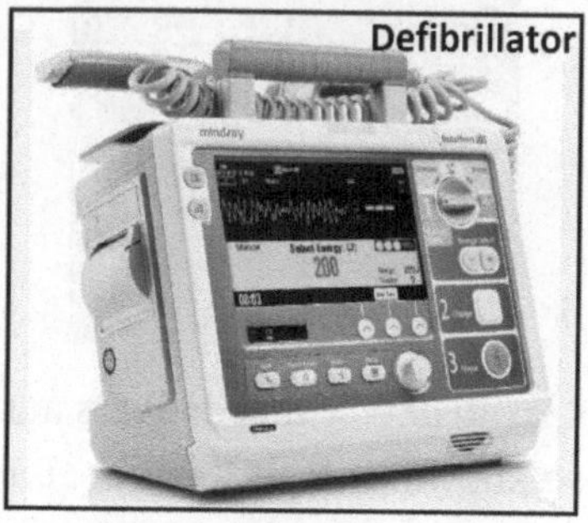

Defibrillator

8. **HFNC (High-Flow Nasal Cannula):** Provides high-flow oxygen, especially for patients with pneumonia.

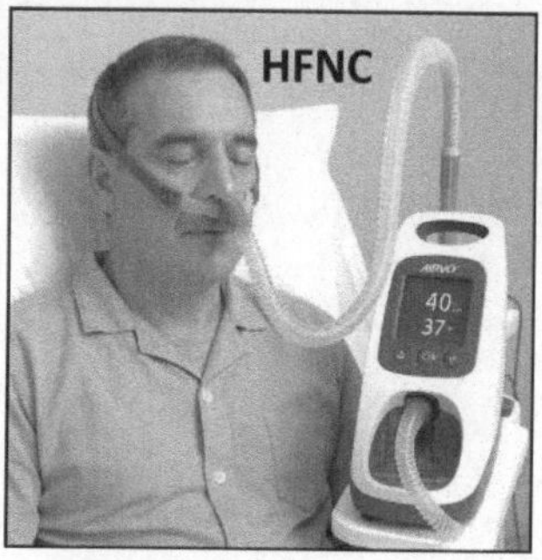

HFNC

9. **SCD (Sequential Compression Device):** Inflates and deflates cuffs tied to the legs to prevent blood clots.

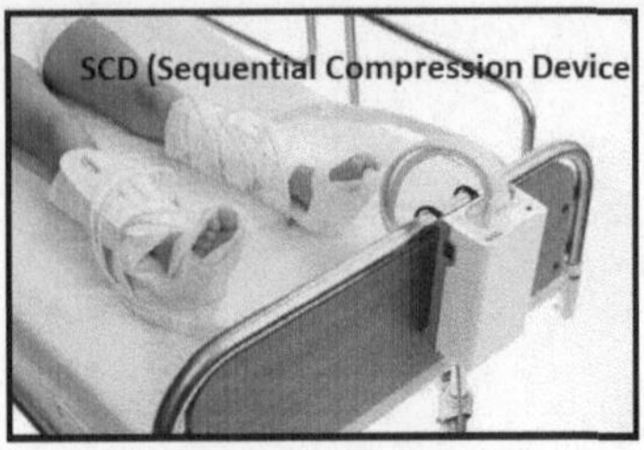

10. **IABP (Intra-Aortic Balloon Pump):** Helps the heart pump blood more effectively. This device is used for patients with low heart pumping capacity for few days when they undergo cardiac procedures or cardiac surgery.

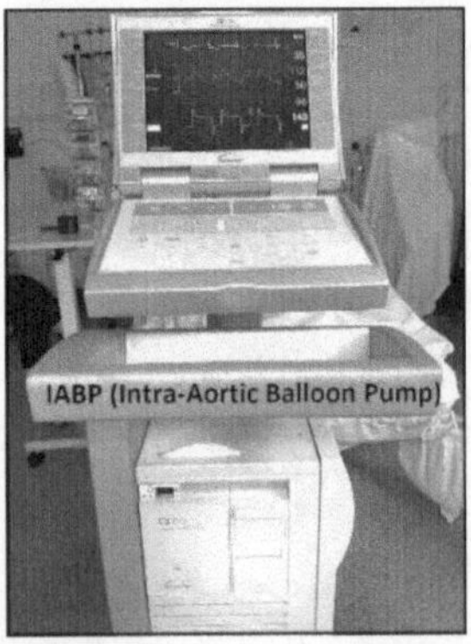

11. **Feeding Pump:** A small device that delivers nutritional liquid through a feeding tube (also known as **Ryle's tube**) at a controlled speed.

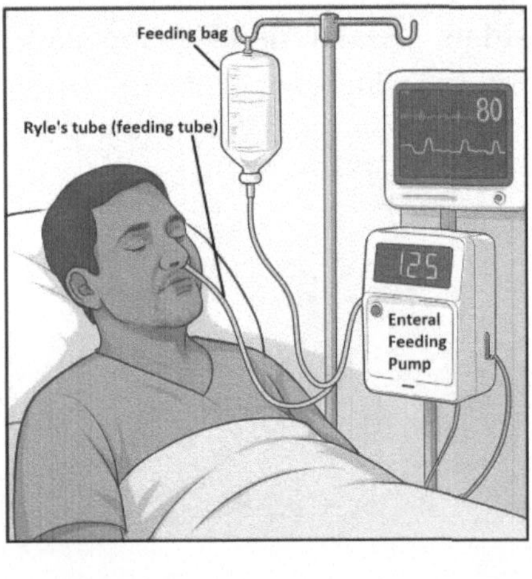

12. **External Pacemaker:** Helps maintain heart rate after a temporary pacemaker is implanted by a cardiologist for the patients with very low heart rate.

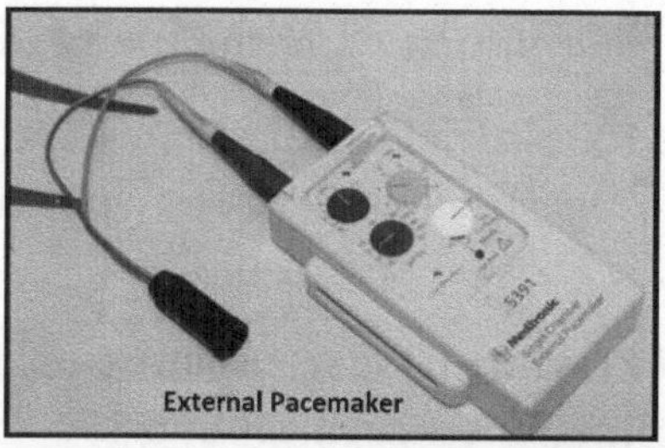

13. **Warmer:** Supplies external heat through a blanket for patients who have chills due to the cold ICU environment.

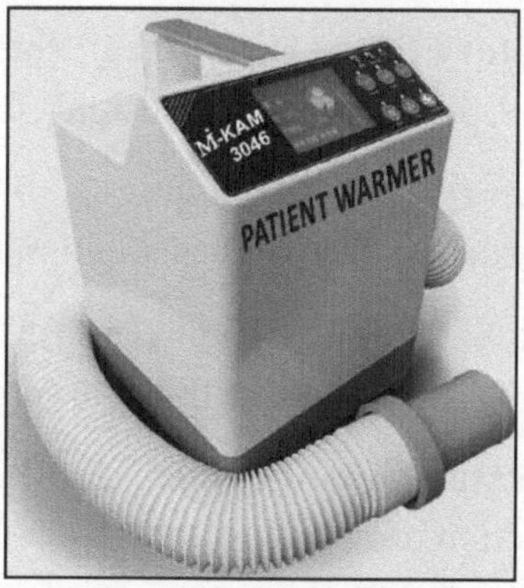

14. **Air Mattress:** Special mattresses like 'Alpha' or 'Nimbus' are used for bed-bound patients to prevent bedsores. Although helpful, these mattresses alone cannot fully prevent pressure sores. Movement and care are also essential.

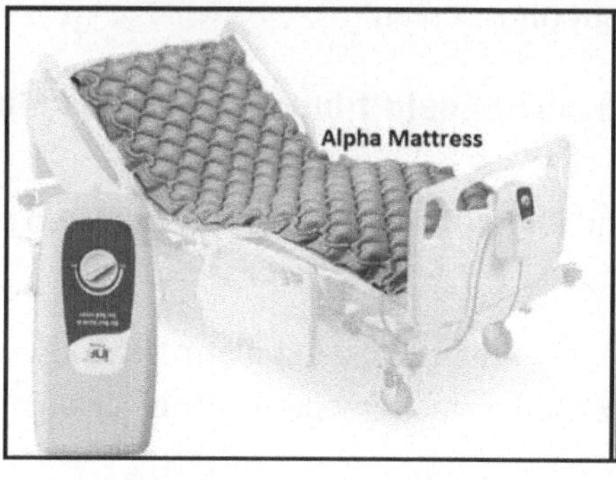

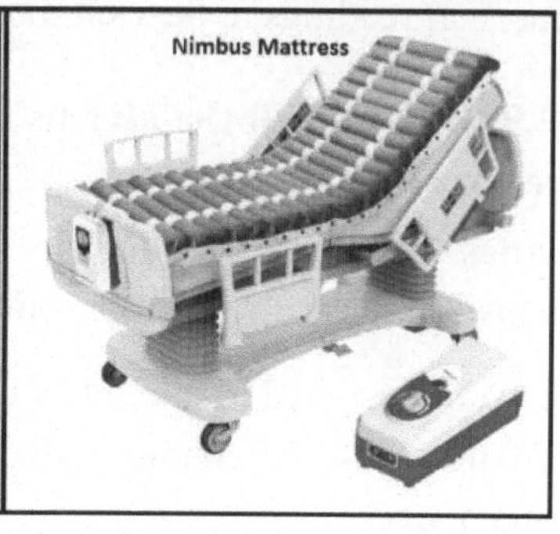

Q2.8: What does it mean if a vital sign is too high or too low?

An abnormal vital sign can signal a health problem:

- **High Heart Rate (Tachycardia):** (Heart rate more than 100) May be due to fever, dehydration, anxiety, or heart issues.
- **Low Heart Rate (Bradycardia):** (Heart rate less than 60) Can result from medications, heart problems, or electrolyte imbalances.
- **High Blood Pressure (Hypertension):** Could be caused by stress, kidney problems, or certain medications.
- **Low Blood Pressure (Hypotension):** May happen due to dehydration, bleeding, infections or heart issues.
- **High Respiratory Rate (Tachypnea):** (breathing rate more than 25) May be a sign of pneumonia, asthma, or anxiety.
- **Low Respiratory Rate (Bradypnea):** (breathing rate less than 14) Can occur due to medications, brain injury, or lung problems.
- **Low Oxygen Saturation (Hypoxemia):** (Spo2 less than 92%) Often caused by pneumonia, asthma, or lung disease.
- **High Temperature (Fever):** (more than 100 Fahrenheit) Usually indicates infection or inflammation.
- **Low Temperature (Hypothermia):** (less than 95 Fahrenheit) May be due to exposure to cold, medications, or certain medical conditions.

The ICU team will carefully evaluate and treat accordingly if any abnormal readings appear on the monitor screen.

Q2.9: What do all the alarms mean? Should I be worried every time one goes off?

Alarms are common in the ICU and may sound frequently, but they do not always mean something is wrong.

They are designed to alert staff to potential issues, but alarms can also go off during routine changes—like sudden movements or brief change in oxygen levels.

If you hear an alarm, stay calm. The medical team monitors them closely and responds appropriately. If you're concerned, feel free to ask the ICU team what the alarm means.

Q2.10: Is there anything I should NOT touch on the equipment?

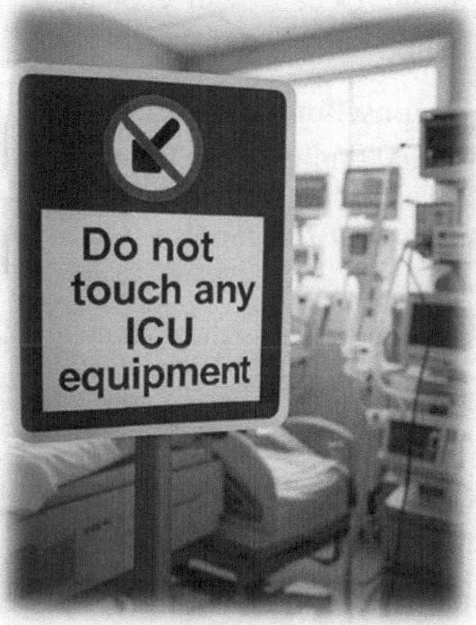

Yes. Do not touch any ICU equipment unless a healthcare professional asks you to.

Tampering with equipment can affect its function and may harm the patient. It also raises the risk of infection.

If you're curious about any device, ask the ICU team—they'll be happy to explain.

Q2.11: What can I expect when someone is admitted to the ICU?

ICU admission can be a stressful time. Here's what usually happens:

- **Initial Assessment:** Doctors and nurses review medical history, perform examinations, and request tests.
- **Monitoring Devices:** The patient is connected to monitors for heart rate, blood pressure, and oxygen levels.
- **Intravenous lines (IV Lines):** Intravenous lines are placed to provide medications, fluids, and nutrition.

- **Catheters:** A urinary catheter may be inserted to drain urine in few patients.
- **Breathing Support:** Oxygen or mechanical ventilation is given if needed.
- **Communication:** Doctors will explain the treatment plan and answer questions.
- **Visiting & Counselling:** The staff will guide you on visiting hours, counselling timings, and ICU policies.

Q2.12: What questions will the medical team ask during the initial assessment?

During the initial assessment, the medical team will ask several questions to understand the patient's medical history and current condition. Be prepared to answer questions about:

- **Past Medical History:** This includes any past illnesses, surgeries, allergies, and medications.
- **Current Medications:** Share a list of all medications the patient is currently taking, including prescription drugs, over-the-counter medicines, and herbal supplements.
- **Allergies:** Inform the medical team about any known allergies, especially to medications or foods.
- **Recent Symptoms:** Describe the symptoms the patient has experienced—such as shortness of breath, chest pain, or fever.
- **Events Leading to Admission:** Explain what happened that led to the patient being admitted to the ICU.

Providing accurate and complete information will help the medical team deliver the best possible care for your loved one.

Q2.13: How can I best prepare to answer these questions?

Being ready to answer the medical team's questions can save time and help them make faster decisions. Here are some helpful tips:

- **Gather Medical Records:** If possible, bring any relevant documents, such as medication lists, allergy details, and previous medical history.
- **Talk to Family Members:** If you're not the primary caregiver, speak to other relatives who may know more about the patient's health background.
- **Make a List:** Prepare a written list of the patient's medications, allergies, and past medical conditions to take to the hospital.
- **Take Notes:** During the counselling session, write down important details to help you remember what was discussed.

Q2.14: How can I, as a family member, best interact with the ICU team?

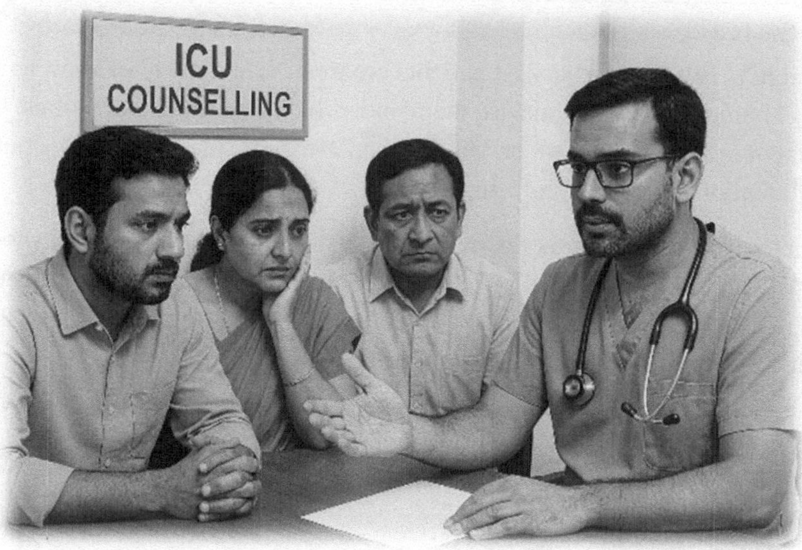

Family members play a valuable role in the ICU care process. Here's how to build a good partnership with the medical team:

- **Introduce Yourself:** Let the team know who you are and that you're a family member.
- **Ask Questions:** Feel free to ask about your loved one's condition, treatment options, and expected recovery.
- **Share Information:** Provide accurate details about your loved one's medical background and current condition.
- **Voice Your Concerns:** Share anything you're worried about and mention what matters most to you and your family.
- **Be Respectful:** Appreciate the team's time, efforts, and expertise.
- **Take Notes:** Write down important points from team discussions so you can refer to them later.
- **Be Patient:** The ICU can be a fast-moving and stressful environment. Trust that the team is working hard to give your loved one the best care possible.

Q2.15: Why are patient's relatives not allowed to stay with the patient in the ICU?

The ICU is where the sickest patients are treated, and many of them have low immunity, which makes them more likely to catch infections. If relatives frequently visit or stay with patients in the ICU, they could unintentionally pass on infections.

That's why ICU entry is restricted and visiting hours are fixed. Visitors must carefully follow the hospital staff's instructions during these visits. Washing hands with antiseptic solution before and after touching the patient is one of the most important rules.

Other reasons for restricted entry include protecting the privacy of other patients, avoiding interference with nursing care, and managing the limited space around each ICU bed.

Q2.16: Is it compulsory for patient's relatives to stay at the hospital while the patient is in the ICU?

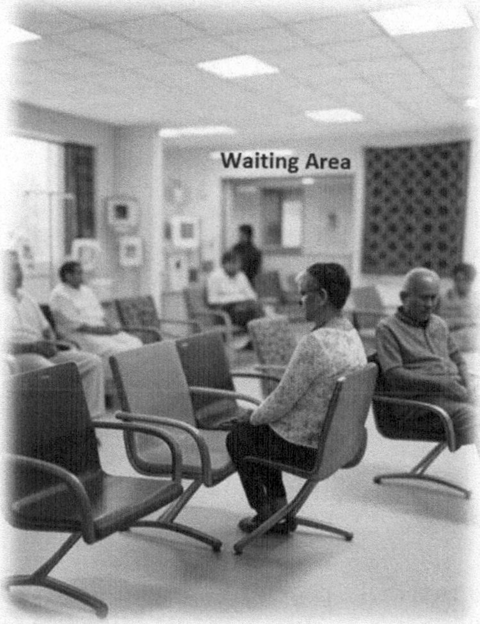

It is not compulsory for patient's relatives to stay at the hospital the entire time the patient is in the ICU.

However, it is recommended that one relative remain near the ICU for some time after admission because doctors may need to speak with them during early counselling sessions to give updates.

Once that initial update is given, relatives can leave if they have other important work. Certain medical procedures require consent from family members, so doctors may ask them to come back to sign forms. Whether to stay in the hospital continuously or not is entirely up to the patient's family.

Q2.17: Why are mobile phones not allowed in the ICU?

Mobile phones are restricted in the ICU to protect the privacy and confidentiality of patient information. Patients should not keep phones with them during ICU treatment because phones can carry germs, and ICU staff cannot be responsible for patients' personal items.

Hospitals may have different rules, and sometimes phones are allowed only for few minutes in special situations—such as making phone call to patient's relative for updates, accessing documents or making payments.

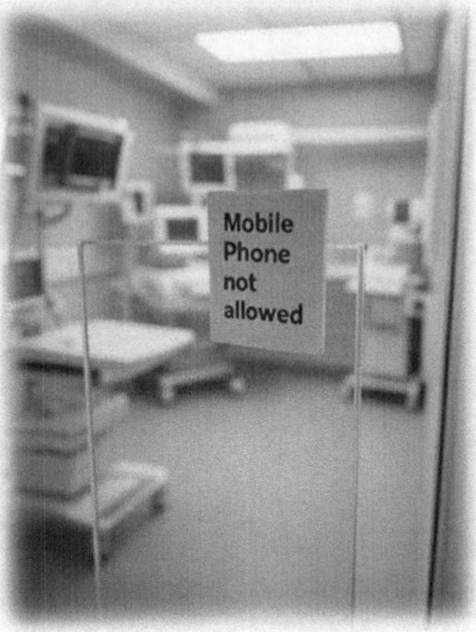

Relatives should never take photos inside the ICU without permission. If they need to photograph a report or document, they must ask the doctor first. Patient records must stay in the hospital, and families should not remove any documents from the ICU without approval.

ICU staff are not responsible for looking after personal belongings, so they usually hand over items like wallets, phones, and jewellery to the patient's relatives. Relatives may be asked to sign a receipt to confirm they've received these valuables.

Q2.18: When will patient's relatives receive the first update after ICU admission?

When a patient is moved to the ICU, relatives can accompany the patient only up to the entrance. Naturally, families feel anxious while waiting outside and may wish to speak to the doctor immediately. It's important to stay calm. The security guard at the ICU entrance may not allow patient's relatives to enter the ICU without doctor's permission.

ICU doctors give the first update only after starting treatment and stabilizing the patient. If the patient is critically ill, the doctor may need more time with the patient before giving updates. Many critically ill patients require procedures like inserting central lines, arterial lines, or dialysis sheaths, which can delay the counselling session.

Relatives should wait in the designated area until the doctor calls them for counselling. If the patient is stable, doctors usually talk to the relatives within the first hour after initiating the treatment. However, if the patient has very low blood pressure or is on a ventilator, the doctor may be busy with emergency care and cannot give updates immediately. In such cases, relatives may need to wait longer—possibly more than an hour—for any information.

Q2.19: How will patient's relatives know what is happening in the ICU?

ICU patients receive care from many specialists— intensivist, doctors from different specialties, nurses, physiotherapists, respiratory therapists, nutritionists, and others. Because of this multidisciplinary care, it's not practical for doctors to give hourly updates. Doctors usually provide updates once they have reviewed and assessed the patient, and they may do this once or twice a day depending on hospital policy.

Some hospitals have fixed counselling hours, during which the doctor meets briefly with family members to share the latest information and answer questions. Families often feel anxious and eager to know more, but they should remember that recovery from critical illness takes time—sometimes days or even weeks.

If there's no update, it often means the patient's condition hasn't changed. If there is a sudden deterioration, doctors will inform the family as soon as they have managed the emergency. Relatives must remain patient while their loved one is being treated in the ICU.

Arguments with staff at the ICU entrance only create more stress for everyone. Doctors need to focus on care rather than frequent updates, so patience and understanding are essential during this time.

Q2.20: How are decisions made regarding my loved one's care?

Decisions about your loved one's treatment are made by the ICU team, led by the intensivist.

- They consider input from other doctors and the patient's values and preferences. Whenever possible, the team will involve both the patient and family members in decision-making.
- If the patient is unable to participate due to medical condition, the doctors will make choices based on what's in the patient's best interest.
- Advance directives—such as written medical preferences—will also be respected if available.

Q2.21: Why don't hospitals allow patient's relatives to bring medicines or injections from outside?

Sometimes patient's relatives ask doctors for permission to buy injections or medicines from outside, but hospitals usually don't allow it for several important reasons.

Hospitals have in-house pharmacies that follow strict safety and quality standards for all medications and injections. If relatives bring medicines from outside, it could put the patient at risk because the hospital cannot guarantee the safety or authenticity of these medicines.

External medicines might be contaminated, expired, or not stored correctly—especially those that require controlled temperatures or special handling. Therefore, all medications needed for treatment should be provided by the hospital's pharmacy.

In rare cases, if a specific medicine is unavailable in the hospital, the staff may ask relatives to procure it from a different hospital or pharmacy. Most routine medicines are available in the hospital's pharmacy, ensuring safety through proper quality control.

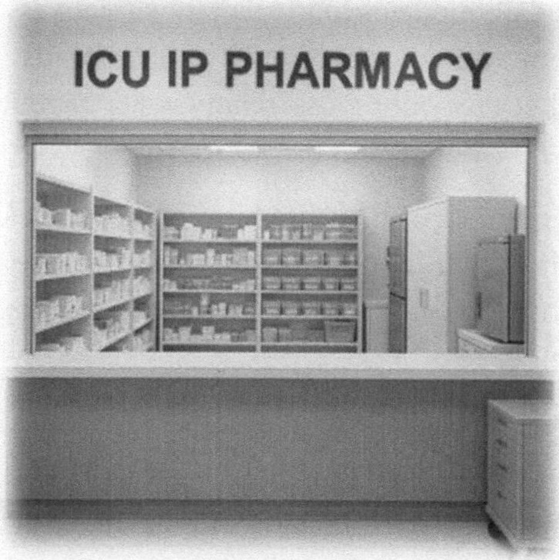

Relatives should not ask permission to buy medicines from outside even if they are cheaper, because compromising patient safety for cost is not advisable. Whenever patient's relatives have such thought, they should ask a simple question to themselves. "Would they bring popcorn from home into a movie theatre that doesn't allow outside food?"

Once a patient is admitted, the hospital is responsible for all tests and medications, and relatives should not request for various investigations at other labs if tests are cheaper there. If the hospital lacks certain equipment, patient can be referred to another facility for that specific investigation.

Q2.22: Why are only a limited number of relatives allowed during the ICU counselling session?

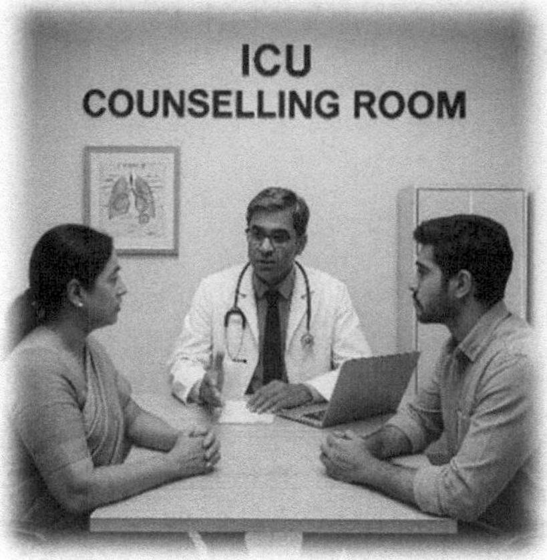

ICU doctors give daily updates to the patient's relatives, and it's easier to explain the patient's condition if only a few family members attend counselling. That's why only close relatives are permitted during these sessions.

Doctors must spend most of their time inside the ICU caring for patients, not in long meetings with families. If too many people are present, they may ask unnecessary questions and take up valuable time that should be spent on patient care.

Doctors cannot meet each family member individually, so all close relatives should be available at once to hear the update. Different hospitals have different policies for visiting hours and counselling sessions.

The ICU is a restricted area, and crowding near the entrance should be avoided. It is hard for security staff to manage large groups of people, so only a few family members are allowed during each session.

Q2.23: Why don't ICU nurses provide detailed information about the patient during visiting hours?

ICU patients need constant monitoring and multiple treatments, and nurses are always busy managing their care. Their main role is to monitor the patient and administer medications. Relatives should not disturb nurses by asking questions while they are actively caring for patients.

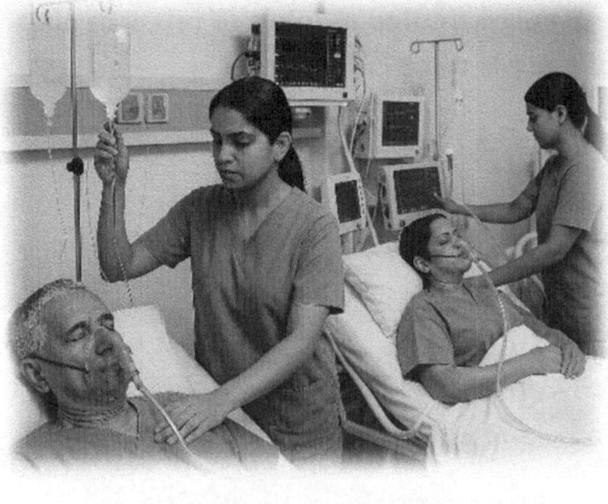

- Although nurses are aware of the patient's condition, they may not answer questions about treatment because they don't want to give incomplete or incorrect information.

- Nurses may not know what the doctor discussed with the family during the counselling session, and they are not responsible for explaining treatment plans.
- Nurses work in shifts and may not know the long-term outcomes because they do not make medical decisions.
- During visiting hours, nurses might be busy in giving some important treatment and they should not get distracted.
- If the patient is unconscious or sleeping, relatives may feel curious even if they've already received updates from doctors. Asking nurses too many questions during busy moments may distract them and result in mistakes.

For these reasons, families should avoid asking nurses about the patient's condition or treatment during visiting hours.

Q2.24: Can ICU doctors allow a short prayer at the bedside for a critically ill patient based on religious beliefs?

If the patient is critically ill and relatives want to say a prayer at the bedside as part of their faith, doctors may allow it—only if it doesn't interfere with treatment.

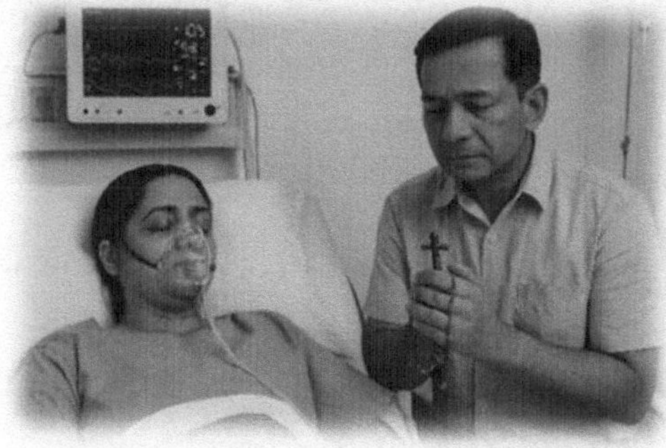

Relatives might also request to place a holy book or item like a rosary near the patient. However, since ICU patients are more prone to infections and surroundings must be clean, doctors may deny permission to place any objects near the patient if patient is very sick.

Any religious activity at the bedside must not affect the patient's care or safety in any way.

Q2.25: How do patients receive bathing and oral hygiene care in the ICU?

ICU patients are connected to many machines, including blood pressure monitors, pulse oximeters, and ECG monitors. They also receive continuous IV fluids and medications, which makes it difficult to allow them to use bathrooms.

Unconscious or ventilated patients cannot move from their bed, so nurses give them a chlorhexidine scrub bath once a day.

For oral hygiene, nurses use antiseptic mouth solutions and help clean the teeth passively. Sometimes, if a patient's condition improves, he or she may be allowed to walk and use the bathroom.

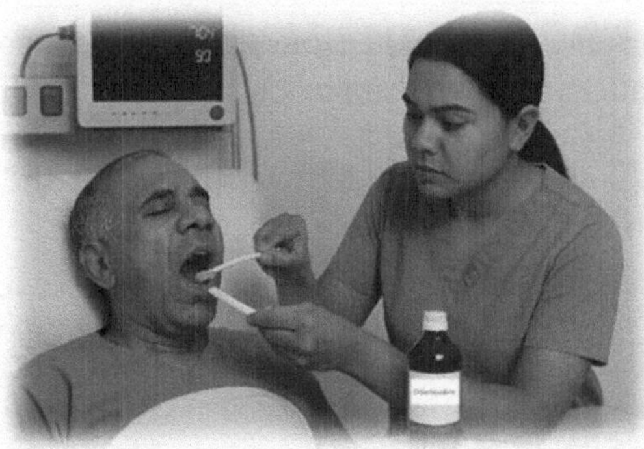

Young patients may feel uncomfortable when they cannot use the washroom normally, but they need counselling to understand that this is for their safety based on their medical condition.

Q2.26: What questions should I ask the medical team during meetings?

Here are some questions you can ask the medical team:

- What is my loved one's current condition?
- What are the goals of treatment?
- What tests have been done, and what were the results?
- What medications is my loved one receiving, and what are their purposes and potential side effects?

- What are the possible complications (unexpected problems) of treatment?
- What is the prognosis (expected recovery and outcome)?
- What can I do to help?
- Are there any decisions that need to be made?

Q2.27: What can I do to support my loved one who is extremely sick?

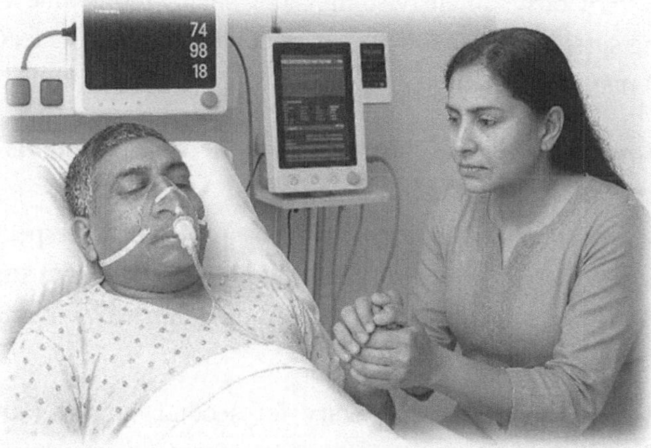

Even if your loved one is unconscious (not awake) or unable to talk, your support can make a difference. Here are some ways to help:

- **Be Present:** Just being near your loved one during visiting hours can provide comfort.
- **Talk to Your Loved One:** Speak in a calm and reassuring voice, even if they can't respond. Share memories, express your love, and give encouraging words.
- **Touch:** Gentle contact, like holding their hand or touching their forehead, can be soothing. (Always sanitize your hands before and after touching the patient.)
- **Take Care of Yourself:** Eat, rest, and take breaks so that you are emotionally and physically strong enough to support your loved one.

Q2.28: How can I get clarification if I don't understand something the medical team is saying?

Don't hesitate to ask for clarification (more explanation) if medical words sound confusing.

You can say: **"I'm sorry, I didn't understand that. Could you please explain it in simpler terms?"** or **"Could you explain this procedure by simple drawing on paper?"**

If ICU is very busy, intensivist may not spend more time during the counselling session but other doctor (someone from the ICU team or other specialist) may answer all other queries and give clarifications if needed.

Q2.29: How can I express my concerns or disagreements with the treatment plan?

If you have concerns or disagree with the plan, speak respectfully and clearly. You can say**: "I'm concerned about…"** or **"I'm not sure I agree with…"** and then explain why. The medical team will listen and try to address your concerns.

If needed, you can request summary for second opinion (advice from another doctor who is not part of the current team).

Q2.30: Which document is necessary to collect from doctors if the patient's relatives want a "second opinion" regarding treatment?

Some patients may need surgery or a procedure as part of their treatment, and relatives may want to confirm this with another trusted doctor before giving consent. To do this, they will need the medical test reports or a short summary from the ICU team. This summary includes the patient's current condition and treatment plan and helps the consulted doctor give guidance. If both the ICU doctor and the family's known doctor suggest the same plan, it helps relatives trust the treatment more.

Getting medical advice from another doctor who is not part of the treating team is called a "**second opinion**." It is perfectly acceptable for relatives to share medical reports to seek another view. Sometimes, this helps the ICU team explain things more clearly, because the known doctor may have already explained the same details.

Hospitals may provide a special document called a **"patient summary"** (brief report about patient's health and treatment), which is usually addressed **"to whom it may concern."** This summary may include many medical terms, and it might be hard for relatives to fully understand all parts.

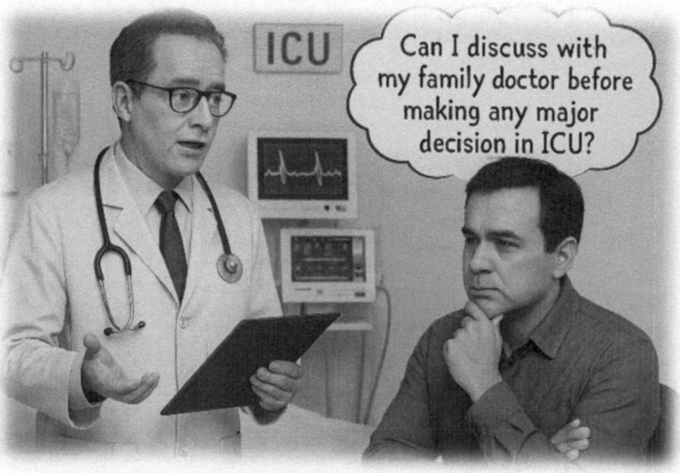
ICU
Can I discuss with my family doctor before making any major decision in ICU?

Relatives sometimes become impatient and keep asking when the summary will be ready. They should understand that ICU doctors may be busy caring for other patients and it may take a few hours to prepare this detailed document. So it is best to wait calmly for medical records or summaries needed for a second opinion.

Q2.31: Why do doctors ask to sign a "LAMA form" (Leave Against Medical Advice) in the ICU?

Not all ICU patients recover completely. Sometimes relatives request discharge from the hospital—either to take the patient to another hospital or back home.

Doctors cannot discharge patients if their condition is still critical or the treatment is incomplete. If relatives insist on discharge despite the risks, it is officially called **"LAMA"**—Leave Against Medical Advice.

A **LAMA form** is a document signed by relatives to take full responsibility when choosing to remove a patient from ICU care during treatment.

LAMA Consent Form

Patient Information

Full Name: ____________

Age / Gender ____________

UHID / IP Number ____________

Date of Admission ____________

Diagnosis: ____________

Ward / ICU: ____________

Reason for Requesting LAMA

☐ Financial constraints ☐ Personal reasons

☐ Dissatisfaction with treatment ☐ Desire for second opinion

Declaration by Patient / Guardian

I ____________ hereby declare that I wish to leave the hospital against the advise of the treating medical team. I understand the risks involved, including potential deterioration of health,complications or death.

- I have been explained the current medical condition
- I am aware that leaving may result in adverse outcomes.
- I absolve the hospital, treating doctors, and staff of any lialbliolity arising from this decision.

Witness Information

Name: ____________

Relationship to Patient ____________

Signature: ____________

Signature of Patient / Guardian

Date & Time: ____________

Physician's Statement

I have explained the risks of leaving against medical advice to the patient/ guardian. They have understood and still wish to proceed.

Physician Name: ____________ Date & Time: ____________

LAMA may be requested by families for the following reasons:

- When relatives are not satisfied with the treatment or hospital
- When they cannot afford ongoing treatment due to financial issues
- When they no longer wish to continue treatment and prefer to take the patient home because of terminal illness or poor outcomes

Relatives should understand that the hospital and its staff will not be responsible for any health issues or emergencies that happen after LAMA discharge.

For example, if a very sick patient dies on the way to another hospital, the original hospital cannot issue a death certificate if the death occurs after LAMA discharge. Even serious events like cardiac arrest (complete cessation of heart beats) can happen during the transfer from ICU to ambulance.

Chapter - 3

Treatments and Procedures in the ICU

Q3.1: What kind of documents are required to be signed by a patient's relatives when the patient is being treated in the ICU?

The **informed consent form** (a permission document explaining risks and procedures) is the most commonly used document in the ICU for many procedures.

Doctors generally explain the procedure to the patient's relatives before performing any **invasive procedures** (procedures that involve entering the body), and the hospital staff always obtains written permission in the form of informed consent.

Here is a list of **common invasive procedures** that may be needed for critically ill patients in the ICU:

1. **Intubation** (placing a breathing tube into the windpipe to support breathing using a ventilator)

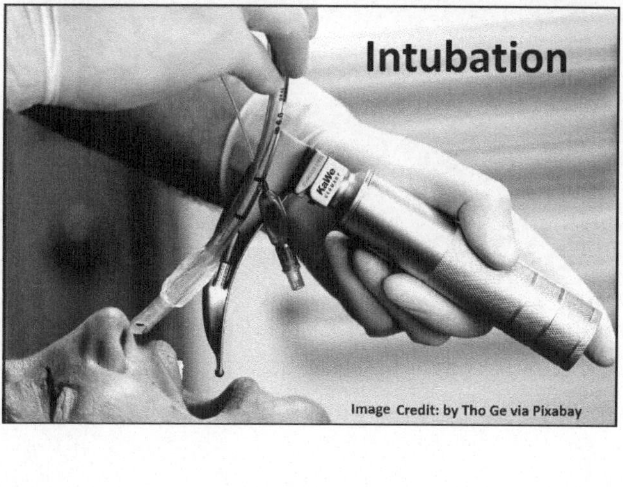

2. **Central line insertion** (placing a catheter into a large vein, usually near the neck or collar bone, to give fluids and medications)

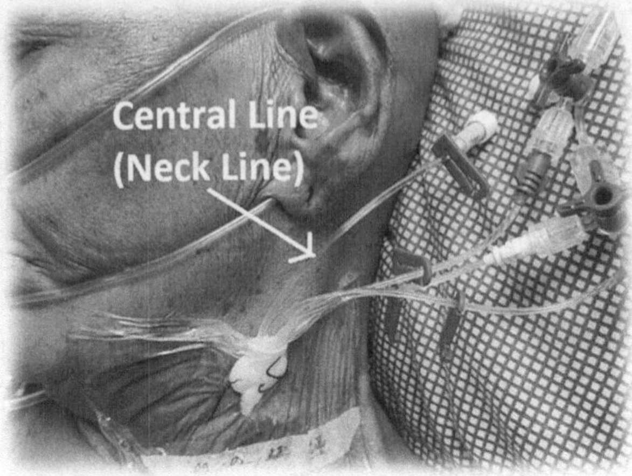

3. **Arterial line insertion** (placing a small catheter near the wrist or groin to monitor blood pressure continuously and collect blood samples for **ABG analysis** [Arterial Blood Gas – checks oxygen, carbon dioxide, and acid levels in the blood])

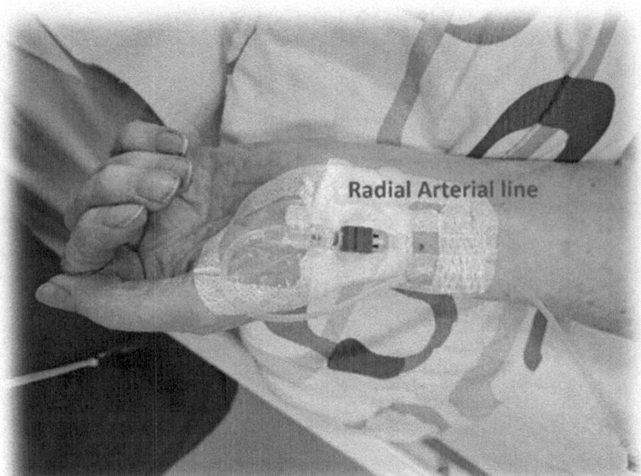

4. **Haemodialysis sheath insertion** (placing a special catheter with ports near the neck or groin to perform dialysis [a process to clean the blood when kidneys are not working])

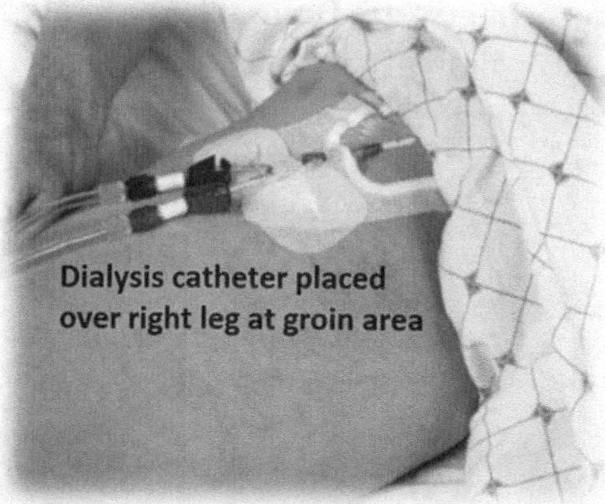

5. **Foley's catheter insertion** (placing a flexible urine tube [made up of silicon or latex material] to measure how much urine is passed hourly)

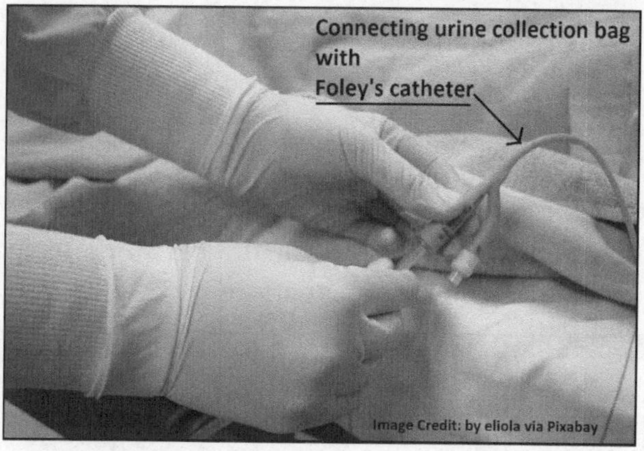

6. **Ryle's Tube insertion** (inserting a feeding tube through the nose or mouth for nutrition or medications which is also known as "Nasogastric-NG tube")

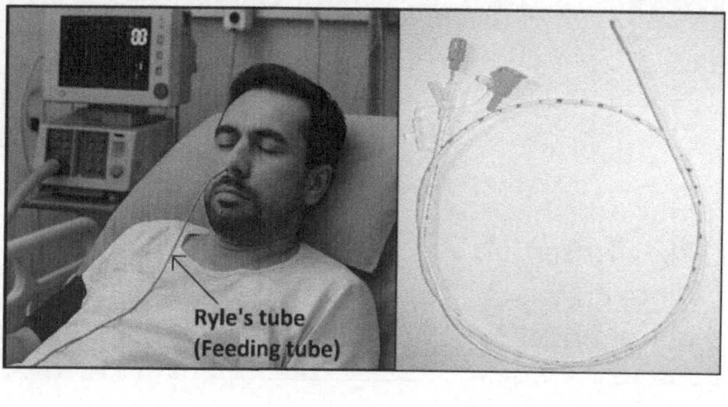

7. **ICD insertion – Intercostal Drain** (placing a tube between the ribs to remove fluid or air from around the lungs)

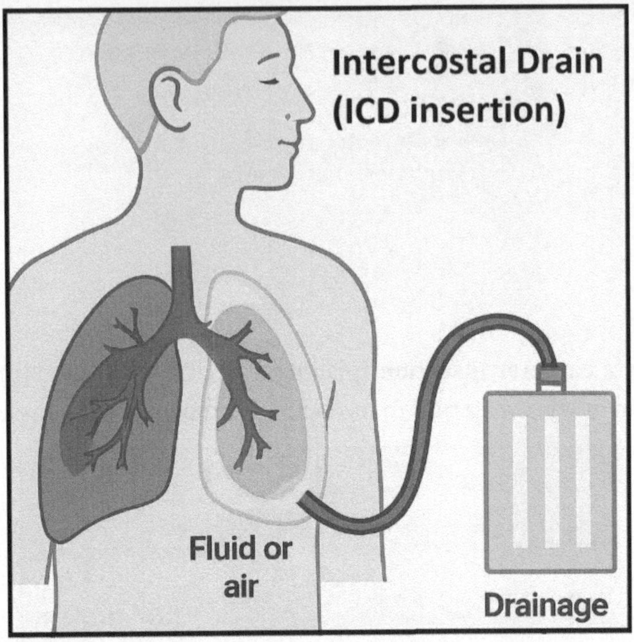

8. **Pig-tail insertion** (placing a small flexible silicon or polyurethane tube to drain fluids from various parts of the body)

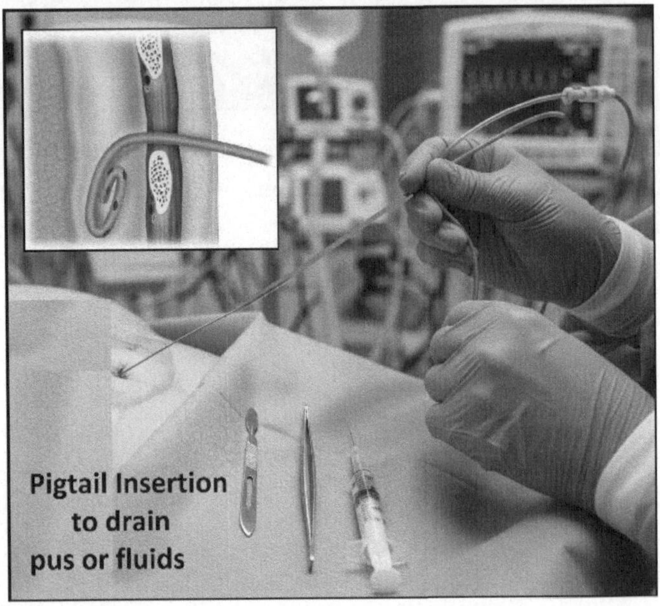

9. **LP – Lumbar Puncture** (introducing a needle in the lower back to collect fluid from around the spinal cord)

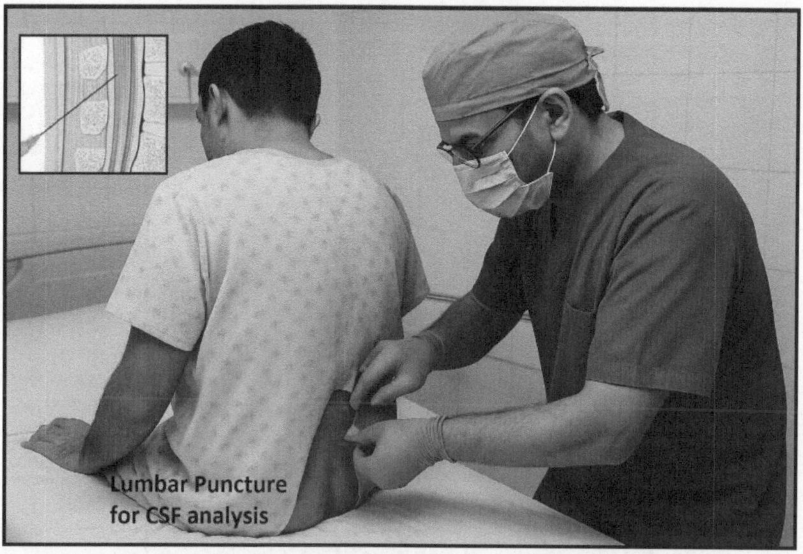

10. **Bone marrow aspiration or biopsy** (using a thick hollow needle to take a sample from inside the hip bone for testing)

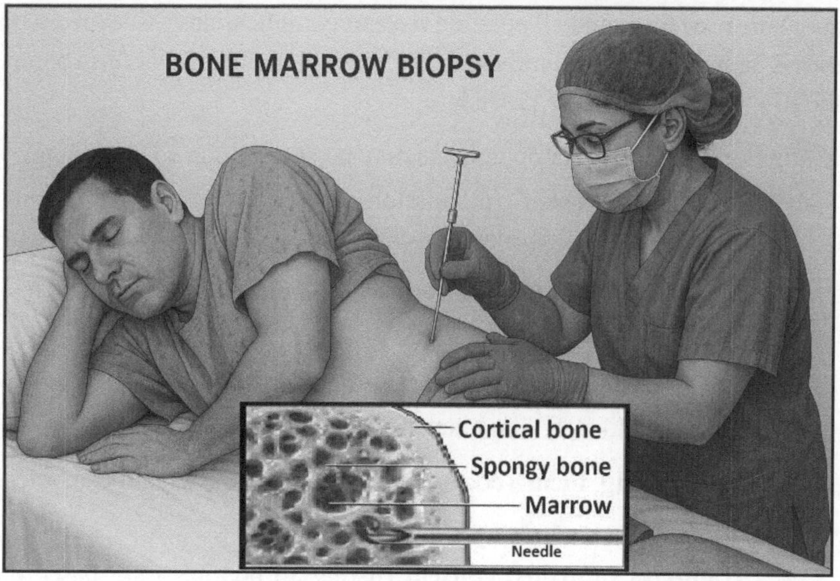

11. **Tracheostomy** (creating an opening in the neck to insert a breathing tube directly into the windpipe)

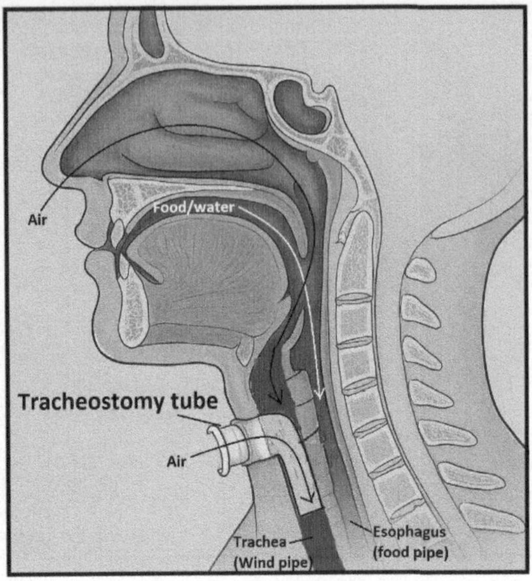

All these procedures require patient's relatives to give permission by signing an informed consent form. The consent form may contain details about the procedure and all possible risks or complications associated with the procedure. Patient's family member has to sign the consent form before the ICU team perform the procedure.

In addition to these, other documents may need to be signed, including:

- **Restraint consent** (permission to safely restrict a patient's movement if they become restless)
- **Blood transfusion consent** (permission to give donated blood to the patient)
- **Viral screening consent** (permission for testing blood for infections like HIV and hepatitis)
- **Counselling form** (documenting discussions with the medical team)
- **High-risk informed consent** (listing all possible risks based on the patient's condition)

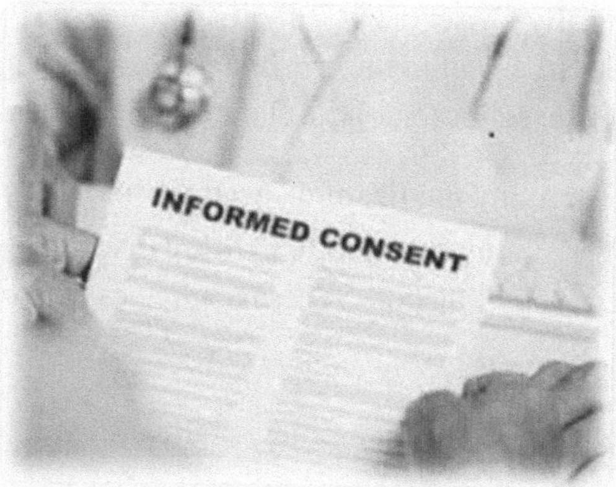

In emergencies, doctors may proceed with life-saving procedures without waiting for prior consent. Sometimes, **informed consent may be waived** (not taken) if there is no time or if the patient cannot communicate and no family member is available.

Q3.2: What is the purpose of the different types of IV lines (intravenous lines)?

Intravenous (IV) lines (tubes that deliver fluids and medications into the veins) are used to give fluids, medicines, and nutrition directly into the bloodstream.

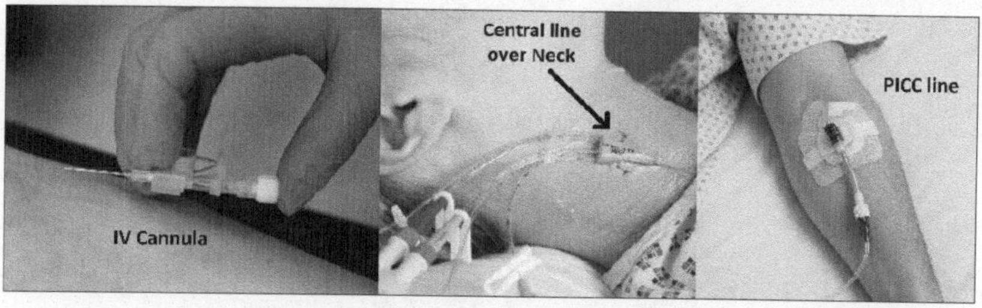

Different types of IV lines are used depending on the patient's condition:

- **Peripheral IV cannula**: A short, thin tube placed into a vein in the arm or hand. It is used for short-term medications or fluids.
- **Central Venous Catheter (CVC)**: A long, thin tube inserted into a large vein in the neck or chest. It is used for long-term treatment and for checking pressure in right side chambers of the heart.

- **Peripherally Inserted Central Catheter (PICC)**: A tube inserted into a vein in the arm, extending to a large vein near the heart. It is used for long-term fluids, medications, or nutrition.

Q3.3: Why are so many medications used in the ICU?

Many medications are used in the ICU to treat various illnesses and to support important body functions. These medicines help to:

- **Treat infections** (using antibiotics)
- **Control pain** (using pain-relieving drugs)
- **Reduce anxiety** (using calming medicines known as sedatives)
- **Support blood pressure** (to raise or lower blood pressure)
- **Control heart rate** (manage heartbeat speed and rhythm)
- **Improve breathing** (to improve lung functions)
- **Prevent blood clots** (stop harmful clot formation)
- **Manage other medical problems** (like diabetes, kidney, and liver conditions)

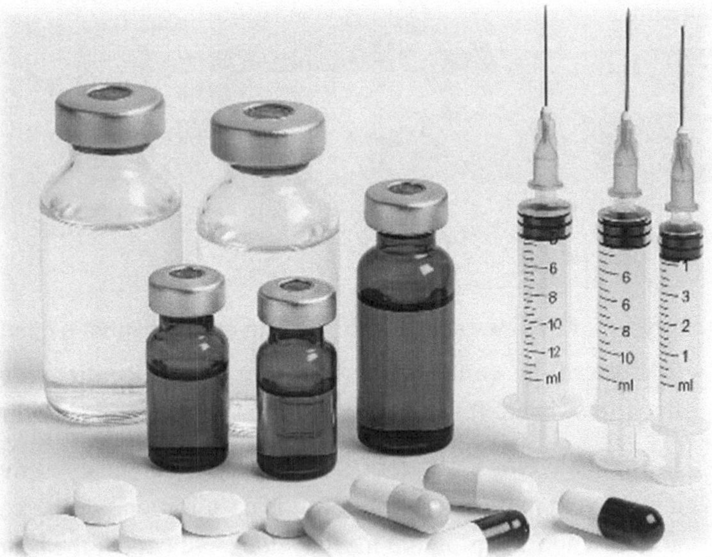

Q3.4: What are some common medications used in the ICU, and what are their purposes?

Here are some commonly used ICU medications:

- **Antibiotics**: To treat infections
- **Pain Medications (Analgesics)**: To relieve pain
- **Sedatives**: To reduce anxiety and help with sleep
- **Vasopressors**: To raise blood pressure
- **Antiarrhythmics**: To correct abnormal heartbeats
- **Bronchodilators**: To open airways and improve breathing
- **Corticosteroids**: To reduce swelling and inflammation
- **Anticoagulants**: To prevent blood clots
- **Insulin**: To control blood sugar levels
- **Diuretics**: To remove excess fluid through excess urine production
- **Proton Pump Inhibitors (PPIs)**: To reduce stomach acid and protect against stomach ulcers

Q3.5: What is sedation, and why is it sometimes necessary in the ICU?

Sedation means using medicines to calm the patient by reducing anxiety, awareness, and restlessness.

It is needed in ICU for several reasons:

- **Promote comfort** (keep patient relaxed and pain-free)
- **Reduce anxiety** (help the patient feel less frightened or agitated)
- **Help medical procedures** (make it easier to perform tasks like inserting a breathing tube or operating machines like ventilators)
- **Support rest and healing** (allow the patient to sleep and recover more effectively)

Q3.6: How are medications administered in the ICU?

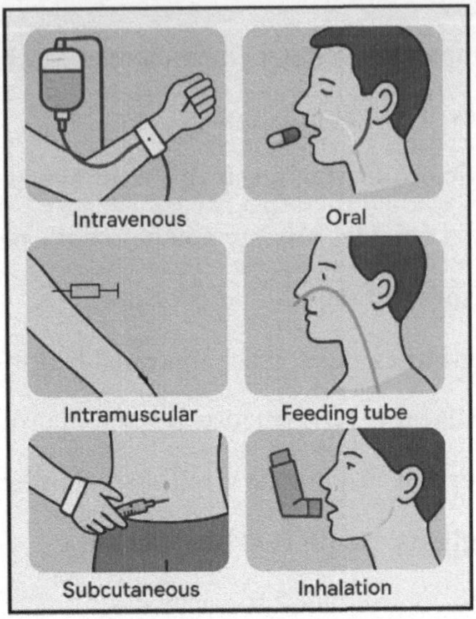

Medications are administered in the ICU using a variety of methods:

- **Intravenous (IV):** Medications are given directly into the bloodstream through an IV line (a tube inserted into a vein).
- **Oral:** Medications are taken by mouth, if the patient is able to swallow.
- **Feeding Tube:** Medications can be given through a feeding tube (a small tube placed through the nose or mouth into the stomach) if the patient cannot swallow.
- **Intramuscular (IM):** Medications are injected into a muscle.
- **Subcutaneous (S/C):** Medications are injected under the skin.
- **Inhalation:** Medications are breathed into the lungs using a nebulizer or inhaler (devices that turn medicine into mist or deliver it directly to the airway).

Q3.7: Why do patients need ventilator support?

Ventilation is the process by which oxygen enters the lungs and carbon dioxide leaves the lungs. When a patient has difficulty breathing, he or she may need breathing support with oxygen or special breathing devices.

There are 2 types of ventilation:

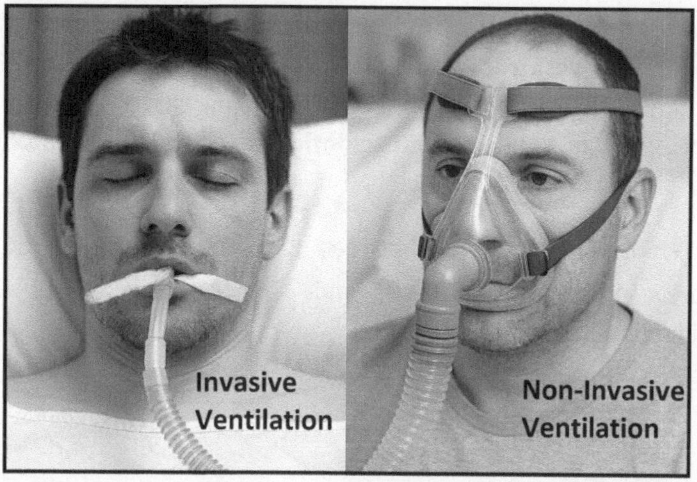

1. **Invasive ventilation:** A tube is inserted into the windpipe (trachea) and connected to a mechanical ventilator (a breathing machine).
2. **Non-invasive ventilation (NIV):** A large clear mask is placed tightly over the face and connected to a bedside NIV machine.

The most common reason for ventilator support is very low oxygen levels (**hypoxia**) due to conditions like:

- **Pneumonia** (lung infection)
- **Heart failure** with fluid in the lungs
- **Airway problems** (issues with breathing tract)

Other reasons include:

1. To remove excess carbon dioxide from the body (common in **COPD** patients—chronic obstructive pulmonary disease from smoking or other causes)
2. To protect the lungs from **aspiration** (when food or fluids enter the lungs), especially if the patient is unconscious
3. To prevent movement during surgeries (ventilator is not required once anaesthesia wears off and patient is conscious after surgery)
4. To give oxygen during **CPR (Cardiopulmonary Resuscitation)** when the patient has no pulse

5. To transport critically ill patients (who may need invasive ventilation for safety during movement)

6. To prevent **respiratory arrest** (cessation of breathing) caused by muscle weakness and severe low blood pressure, especially if the patient has fast and shallow **acidotic breathing** (a breathing pattern due to high acid levels in the body)

Q3.8: What is the difference between a ventilator and BiPAP/CPAP?

All three—**Ventilator**, **BiPAP**, and **CPAP**—are used to support breathing, but they work differently:

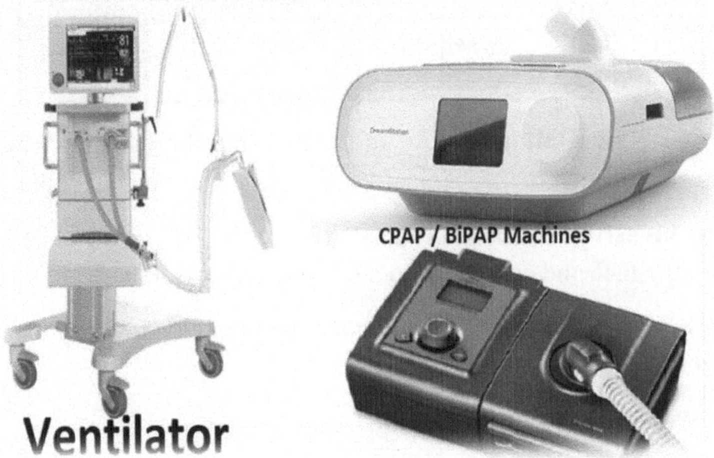

Ventilator: A machine that completely takes over breathing. A tube is inserted into the windpipe (**trachea**) and the ventilator supplies air and oxygen to the lungs. This is used when patients cannot breathe well on their own.

BiPAP (Bilevel Positive Airway Pressure): A non-invasive machine that delivers air through a mask covering the nose and mouth. It gives two pressures—higher pressure while breathing in and lower pressure while breathing out—to help improve oxygen level and ease breathing.

CPAP (Continuous Positive Airway Pressure): A non-invasive machine that gives a constant level of air pressure through a mask. It keeps airways open and helps improve oxygen levels. It is often used for **sleep apnea** (a condition with pauses in breathing during sleep) or mild breathing problems.

Q3.9: Will my loved one be able to talk with all the equipment attached?

Whether your loved one can speak depends on the type of equipment being used:

- **Ventilator:** If a tube is placed in the windpipe (**trachea**), they cannot talk because the tube passes through the vocal cords (voice box).
- **BiPAP/CPAP:** If wearing a tight NIV mask, they may be able to talk—but it might be uncomfortable or difficult.
- **Other Equipment:** Devices like heart monitors, IV pumps, and **arterial lines** (used to check blood pressure) do not affect speech.

If your loved one cannot talk, they can still communicate using methods like:

- Writing notes
- Using hand signals
- Using a communication board (a tool with letters, pictures, or words)

Q3.10: What are the different ways by which a patient can receive oxygen therapy?

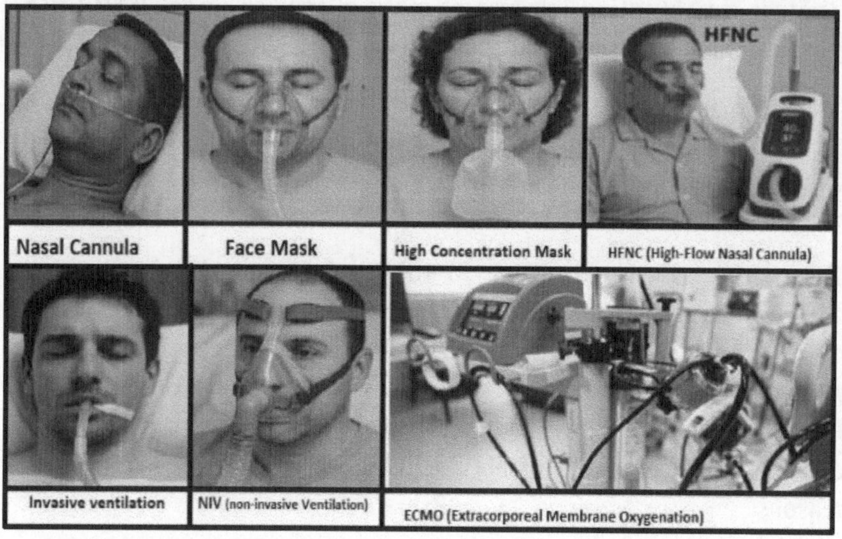

Whenever a patient has low **SpO_2 levels** (oxygen saturation level measured using a **pulse oximeter**—a small device placed on the finger; normal range is 95–100%), doctors advise oxygen therapy.

There are **various devices** used to provide oxygen support:

1) Oxygen Nasal Cannula: This is a transparent tube with two small prongs placed in the nostrils and wrapped around the head. It is used when very minimal oxygen support is required. This method is comfortable because the patient can talk, eat, and drink without disturbing oxygen delivery.

2) Oxygen Face Mask: This is a simple mask used when continuous high oxygen support—up to 15 litres per minute—is needed. It is commonly used in hospitals.

3) High-Concentration Mask: This mask includes a transparent reservoir bag attached to the face mask. It delivers higher oxygen concentration and is used when very high oxygen support is necessary.

4) HFNC (High-Flow Nasal Cannula): An advanced oxygen system that delivers oxygen at a high flow—up to 60 litres per minute. It is especially helpful for patients with **severe pneumonia** (serious lung infection).

5) NIV (Non-Invasive Ventilation): If oxygen levels are not maintained with the devices mentioned above, a patient may need NIV support. This involves a tight-fitting transparent mask connected to a **CPAP/BiPAP** machine (breathing support machines placed beside the bed).

6) Invasive Ventilation (After Intubation)**:** If oxygen levels do not improve, the patient may need **intubation** (placing a tube into the windpipe) and connection to a **mechanical ventilator** (a machine that helps with breathing).

7) ECMO (Extracorporeal Membrane Oxygenation): A highly advanced life-support system used when oxygen levels are not maintained even with maximum ventilator support. Blood passes through a membrane that adds oxygen and removes carbon dioxide. ECMO acts like **artificial lungs**, used until the patient's lungs recover. ECMO is very costly therapy and every patient is not suitable for ECMO due to bleeding risk or other reasons.

Q3.11: How do patients receive food when they are on ventilator support?

Feeding is an important part of ICU care. Patients who are awake and able to swallow can eat meals prescribed by the nutritionist.

Patients who are semi-conscious or unconscious cannot swallow properly. They are fed through a feeding pipe inserted through the nose, called a **Ryle's tube** (a soft tube placed into the stomach through nose or mouth).

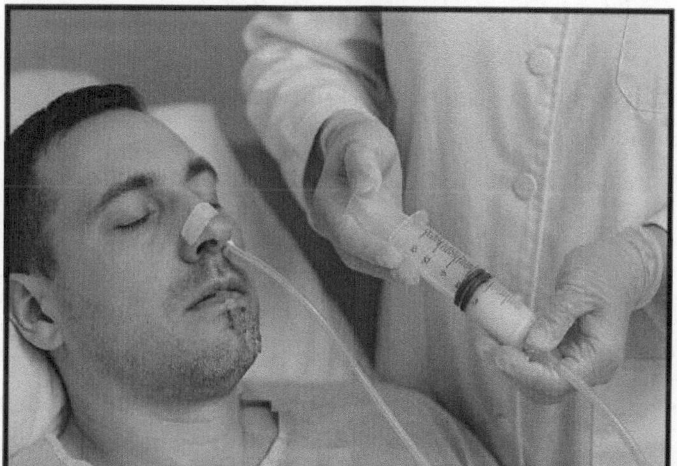
Patient receiving feeds through Ryle's tube (feeding tube)

This method allows liquid nutritional supplements to enter the stomach directly. It avoids the **oropharynx region** (part of the throat), reducing the risk of **aspiration** (when food or liquids mistakenly enter the lungs).

Aspiration can happen during swallowing if the patient is not fully alert or if swallowing muscles are weak. It can also occur with unconscious patients during vomiting when stomach contents go into the lungs.

Nutrition in the ICU is treated as important as medicines. Most patients receive formula feeds containing carbohydrates, fats, proteins, micronutrients, and fluids. Daily calorie needs are calculated, and supplements are adjusted accordingly.

In a few cases—such as after major intestinal surgeries—patients may be fed using **TPN (Total Parenteral Nutrition)**, which is liquid nutrition given directly into the bloodstream to avoid using the digestive system.

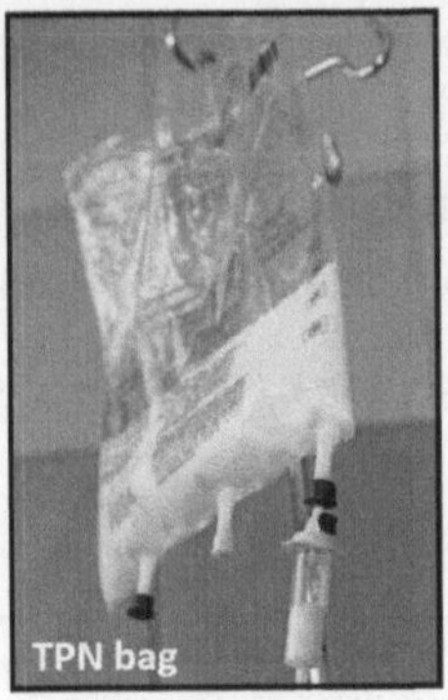

Q3.12: Why do patients develop significant swelling all over the body while in the ICU?

Patients treated in the ICU may develop swelling (medically called **edema**) in one area—like the face, legs, or hands—or throughout the body (called **anasarca**).

Critically ill patients need complete bed rest and cannot move. Without limb movement, fluids can collect in soft tissues, causing swelling.

Doctors refer to swelling in the legs or hands as **dependent edema**. This usually improves once the patient starts moving again.

Even healthy people may notice swelling in feet after long travel by bus, car or aeroplane without walking—similarly, ICU patients may have swelling in feet, legs, palms, and arms due to immobility.

Other causes include:

- **Thrombophlebitis** (swelling and redness at the IV cannula site due to inflammation)
- **Venous congestion** (pressure build-up) causing a swollen tongue or lips in ventilated unconscious patients
- **Fluid leakage** from an **intravenous cannula** (a small catheter placed in vein) causing temporary swelling at cannula site

When swelling affects the entire body (**anasarca**), it may be due to:

- **Heart problems** (poor pumping capacity of the heart)
- **Kidney failure** (fluid not removed effectively out of the body)
- **Low albumin levels** (protein deficiency)

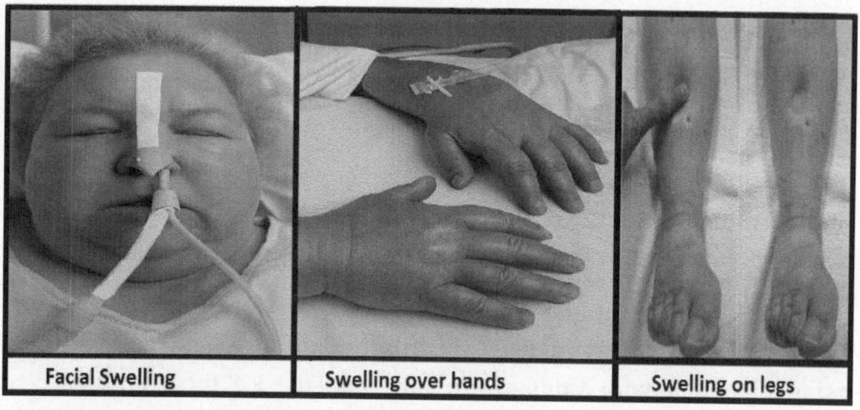

Treatment may include:

- **Diuretics** (medicines that increase urine output) for heart patients
- **Dialysis** (blood filtering) for kidney patients

Q3.13: Why do patients need dialysis even when they have adequate urine output?

Dialysis is a process where the patient's blood passes through a **dialysis machine**—filtering out toxins and acid—and returns clean to the body.

Families easily understand dialysis when urine output is absent. But confusion arises when patients pass urine yet are advised dialysis.

It's important to understand that dialysis is advised for multiple reasons. Even with **normal urine output**, dialysis may be needed due to:

- **Very high potassium levels** (called **hyperkalemia**, which affects heart function)
- **Very high urea levels** causing brain problems (**uremic encephalopathy:** excess sleepiness)
- **Fluid overload** causing difficulty in breathing (**pulmonary edema:** excess water accumulation in the lungs)
- **Persistent high acid in blood (refractory acidosis)**
- **Heart inflammation due to high urea** (**uremic pericarditis**)
- **Poison ingestion** (certain toxins can be removed via dialysis)
- **Chronic kidney disease** (long-term poor kidney function)

Even if the patient is urinating, dialysis may still be essential to clear toxins, balance electrolytes, and support vital organs.

Q3.14: Why do patients need tracheostomy?

Trachea means the windpipe (airway between the lungs and mouth through which breathing occurs), and **tracheostomy** is a procedure where a small breathing tube is inserted into the trachea by creating a hole in the middle of the neck.

When a patient needs **invasive ventilator support** (assisted breathing using a machine with a tube) for a long time, the **ET tube** (endotracheal tube—long breathing tube placed through the mouth) is replaced by a **tracheostomy tube** (short breathing tube placed through the neck) through this procedure.

For example, if a patient has severe **pneumonia** (lung infection) and requires ventilator support for more than 5–6 days without adequate lung recovery, a tracheostomy becomes necessary for prolonged ventilation.

Keeping an ET tube in place for more than a week can cause **subglottic stenosis** (narrowing of the windpipe below the vocal cords due to pressure), which may lead to breathing difficulty after the ET tube is removed.

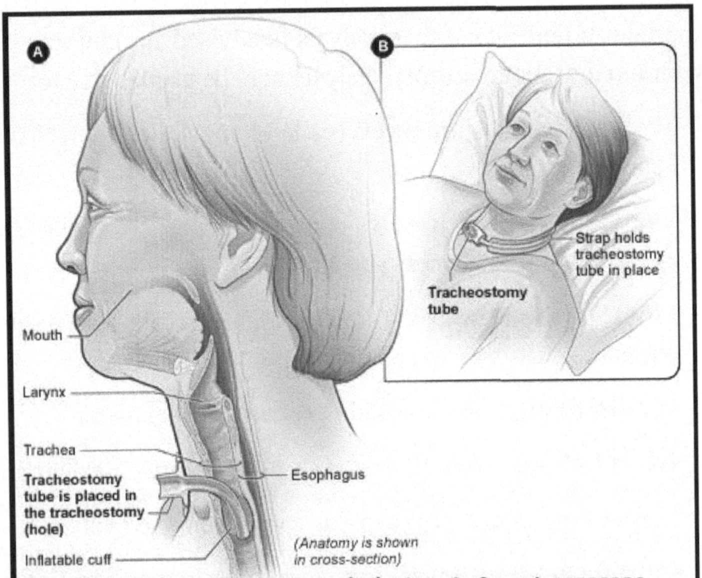

https://commons.wikimedia.org/w/index.php?curid=29588234

Benefits of tracheostomy for prolonged ventilator support include:

- Breathing through a short tube is easier than a long tube.
- Less risk of tube bending or kinking due to its short and firm design.
- Easier to clean by regular suctioning, reducing blockage compared to ET tubes.
- Patient can be quickly disconnected and reconnected to the ventilator when needed.
- Mouth is free from tubes, making it more comfortable.
- Easier to move out of bed and walk with a tracheostomy tube.

Sometimes, even if the lungs are healthy, patients may need a ventilator for other reasons—such as **stroke** (brain attack), **brain infection**, **head injury** from an accident, or **cardiac arrest** (during resuscitation). In these cases, the endotracheal tube or tracheostomy tube helps prevent **aspiration** (entry of food or fluid into the lungs).

Since neurological conditions take time to recover, patients with serious brain issues need tracheostomy until improvement. If ventilated patients remain **semi-conscious** or **unconscious** for over 5–6 days, tracheostomy helps in the process of **weaning** (gradual reduction of ventilator support).

Q3.15: Why do patients need bronchoscopy?

Bronchus is the airway that branches from the trachea and carries air into the lungs.

Bronchoscopy is a procedure in which a **videoscope** (tiny camera tube) is inserted into the bronchus to clean airways and collect **mucus samples** (fluid from lungs) for lab testing in cases like pneumonia. Sometimes, bronchoscopy is needed repeatedly when **mucus plugs** (thick mucus blocking airways) form often.

Apart from cleaning secretions and mucus plugs, bronchoscopy is also useful to take biopsy (small piece of tissue) in certain clinical conditions.

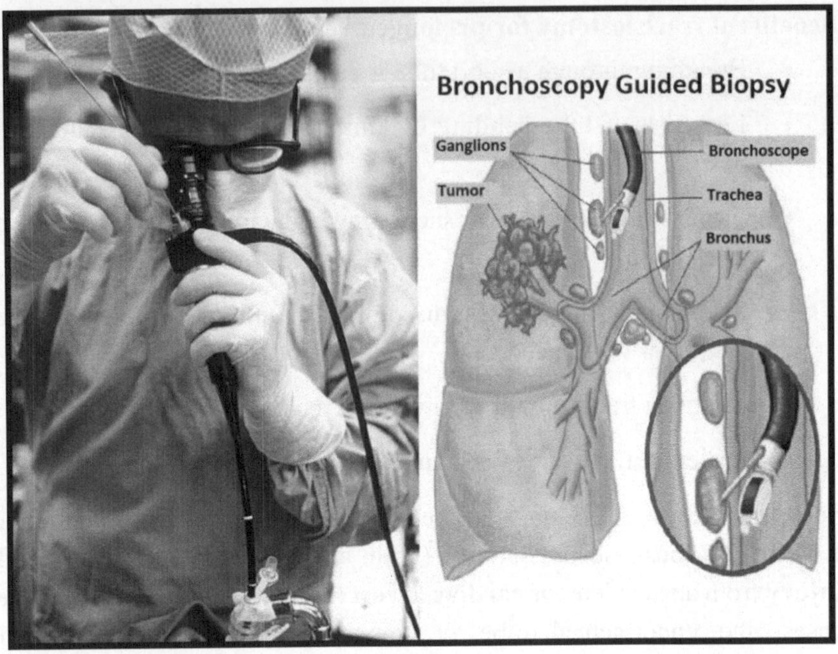

In awake patients, a **bronchoscope** (small pipe with camera) is inserted through one nostril while using **local anaesthetic spray** (medicine to make the procedure pain-free). The scope passes through the vocal cords into the trachea, and suction is used to clear mucus from the major bronchus and branches. These secretions are sent for microbiological tests to detect bacteria or viruses, helping doctors choose the right medicine.

If a patient is already **intubated** (breathing tube in windpipe) and on a ventilator, the bronchoscope is passed through the ET tube and samples are taken during **lavage** (washing the airway with fluid). After the procedure, the patient is reconnected to the ventilator.

Bronchoscopy is common in patients needing long-term ventilator support, as they are more prone to **lung collapse** or **blocked airways**. It may also be used to stop **bleeding** in the lungs or help with intubation in cases of **difficult airway anatomy** (unusual throat or windpipe structure).

Q3.16: Why do patients need endoscopy?

Endoscopy means using a videoscope to look inside the body.

Different types of endoscopy include:

- **Nasal endoscopy:** For the nose.
- **UGIE (Upper Gastrointestinal Endoscopy):** For the esophagus (food pipe), stomach, and duodenum (part of the small intestine).
- **Colonoscopy:** For the colon (large intestine), to find reason for blood in stools or to screen for colon cancer in older adults.

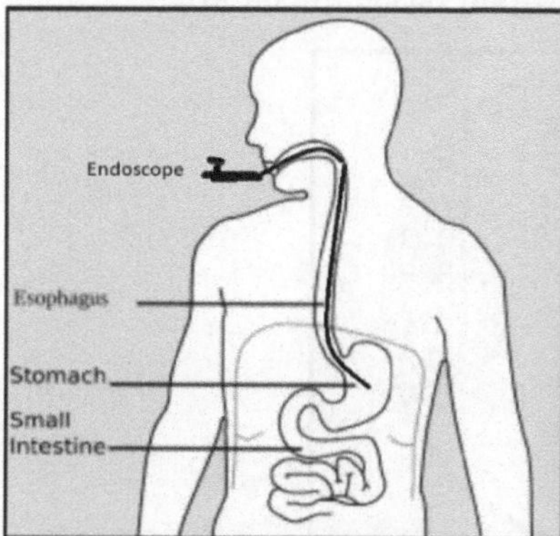

Upper Gastro-intestinal Endoscopy

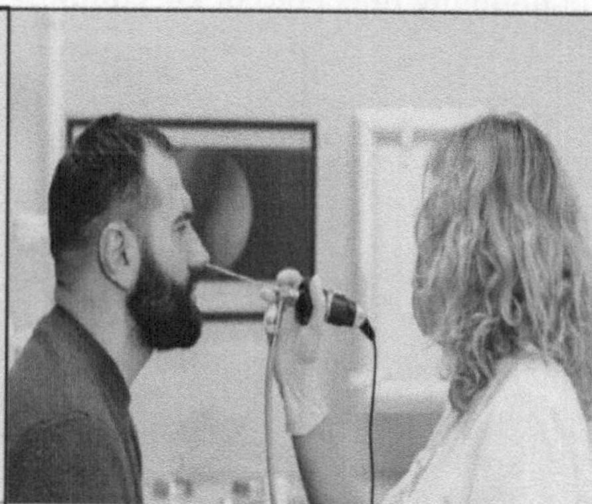

Nasal Endoscopy

UGIE helps detect bleeding, ulcers, or growths in the food pipe or stomach and is advised in situations such as:

- Vomiting blood (known as **hematemesis** – fresh or dark brown)
- Black stools (known as **melena** – dark or tar-like stool)
- Low haemoglobin levels (**anaemia**)
- Difficulty swallowing
- Patients with **chronic alcoholism** (to check for bleeding spots in the food pipe)
- Stomach pain before or after eating (to check for **ulcers**)
- Swallowed objects (e.g., coins, fish bones)
- **Jaundice** [yellowing of skin and eyes] to establish free bile flow

Some patients may receive mild sedation or pain relieving medications during endoscopy or colonoscopy.

Q3.17: Why do patients need lumbar puncture?

Lumbar puncture (LP) is a bedside procedure often needed in the ICU.

A **thin needle** is inserted into the lower back to collect **CSF (Cerebrospinal Fluid)**—a clear fluid that surrounds the brain and spinal cord. This procedure is done when a patient has **altered sensorium** (confused behaviour or reduced consciousness), to test for **meningitis** (brain lining infection) or **encephalitis** (brain tissue infection).

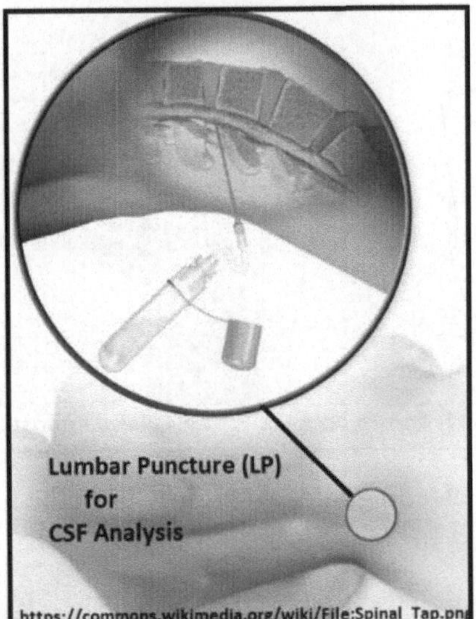

https://commons.wikimedia.org/wiki/File:Spinal_Tap.png

Collected CSF is sent for lab testing to check for viruses or bacteria. Doctors may explain possible risks like **bleeding**, **infection**, or **headache**. To reduce bleeding risk, doctors check **platelet count** (blood clotting cells) and **INR** (International Normalized Ratio—a blood clotting test) before the procedure.

Lumbar puncture usually takes 10–15 minutes and is done with the patient lying on their side or sitting up. Families often worry about pain, but the needle is very thin and does not cause significant discomfort. There is no association between this procedure and **chronic back pain** in the future.

Some **neurological diseases** are diagnosed through CSF testing, and in cases of **hydrocephalus** (excess fluid in the brain), CSF drainage itself becomes part of the treatment.

Q3.18: Why do doctors advise 'culture reports' more often for patients in ICU?

Culture and sensitivity tests (lab tests used to detect infections) help identify bacteria or other microbes in samples like **blood**, **urine**, **pus**, **tissue**, or other body fluids.

When a patient with signs of infection—such as **fever**—is admitted to the ICU, doctors often collect samples based on symptoms and start antibiotics. These samples are sent to the **microbiology lab** for culture testing, and results are typically ready in 2–3 days.

Sometimes doctors need to change antibiotics after reviewing the results of this test, which helps treat the infection faster. If the patient doesn't improve, the test may be repeated.

Relatives should understand that culture tests may take over 2–3 days to identify bacteria or other organisms.

Doctors may also use **Multiplex PCR** (Polymerase Chain Reaction—a rapid test to detect bacteria, viruses, or infections in one sample) for faster diagnosis. Some doctors prefer traditional culture tests alone, while others request both PCR and culture tests for accuracy.

Q3.19: Why do doctors advise daily blood tests when the patient is treated in ICU?

Several blood tests are monitored daily in ICU patients, especially:

- **CBP (Complete Blood Picture)** – checks red and white blood cells and platelets
- **Creatinine** – assesses kidney function
- **Electrolytes** – checks **sodium**, **potassium**, and **chloride** levels

TLC (Total Leukocyte Count) and **platelet count** may fluctuate based on infection severity, so CBP and kidney function tests (creatinine, urea and electrolytes) are done daily.

Critically ill patients often have vital changes that affect organ function, so **liver** and **kidney** tests are done regularly.

If patients have breathing problems or kidney issues, doctors may do **ABG (Arterial Blood Gas)** tests frequently to measure oxygen, carbon dioxide, and acid level in blood.

To collect blood samples, nurses may need to prick the arm, which can cause minor bruising or skin marks. If the patient has a **central line** or **arterial line** (special tubes placed in large veins or arteries), blood can be drawn directly without repeated pricks. Prolonged ICU treatment may lead to low **haemoglobin** (red blood cell levels), partly due to frequent sampling.

Each test provides useful information and helps guide treatment. Relatives should know that all ICU tests are clinically relevant; doctors do not advise unnecessary blood tests.

Q3.20: Why do doctors stop anti-diabetic tablets and start insulin injections in ICU?

Anti-diabetic medicines are also called **OHAs (Oral Hypoglycaemic Agents)**. Relatives often ask why these tablets are stopped in ICU—it's a valid question with a scientific reason.

When the patient is critically ill and eating less or not at all, OHAs can lower blood sugar too much, leading to **hypoglycaemia** (very low sugar causing sweating, confusion, or unconsciousness). To prevent this, tablets are stopped, and blood sugar is controlled using short-acting **insulin injections**.

If the patient has low **blood pressure**, medicine absorption from the stomach becomes poor, so most medications are given by injection during critical illness. Once the patient improves, injectable medicines can be switched back to tablets before moving out of ICU.

Alongside anti-diabetic tablets, other medicines may also be stopped. For example, medicines causing **drowsiness** are withheld if the patient has **neurological problems**, so doctors can monitor consciousness.

Relatives should not worry about daily medications being withheld during ICU care. After recovery, the patient may restart their previous medicines upon discharge.

Q3.21: Why do many patients suddenly accumulate water in the lungs (Pulmonary Edema)?

Lungs are sponge-like organs that support breathing by exchanging oxygen and carbon dioxide. Tiny lung cavities called **alveoli** may fill with water if there is high **blood pressure** or **fluid overload**. This impairs gas exchange and causes breathing difficulty with low oxygen levels. This condition is called **Pulmonary Edema** (swollen lungs with water).

- Pulmonary edema is common in patients with **heart issues**—especially poor pumping capacity of heart or high blood pressure.
- Patients with **kidney failure** may not produce enough urine, causing fluid accumulation, which may also lead to pulmonary edema.
- It may occur after **multiple blood transfusions** or **IV fluids**.
- Rarely, it can happen after draining excess lung fluid (**pleural effusion**) and is then called **re-expansion pulmonary edema**.
- **Negative pressure pulmonary edema** may occur if a patient breathes forcefully against a blocked airway—like swelling near the **vocal cords (laryngospasm)**.

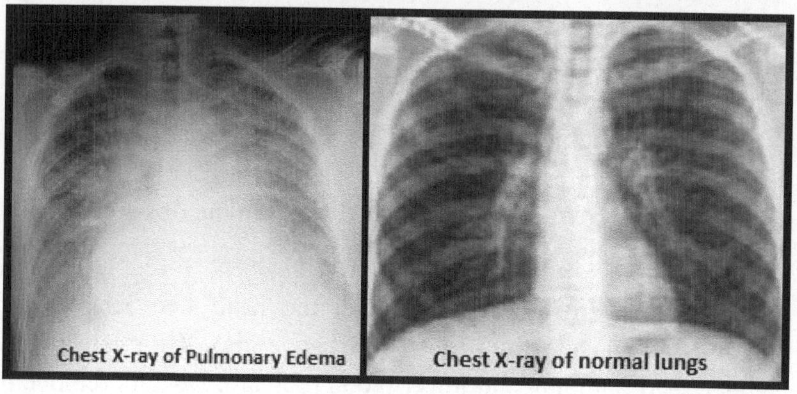

Treatment includes:

- **Diuretics** (injections or tablets to increase urine output and remove extra fluid from the body)
- **Positive pressure ventilation** using **NIV (Non-Invasive Ventilation)** or **invasive ventilation**

If medications and NIV do not help, **intubation** (inserting a breathing tube in wind pipe and connecting to a ventilator) may be needed. Relatives should understand that ventilator support is not only used for pneumonia—it can be life-saving in many other critical conditions, including pulmonary edema.

Q3.22: Why do some patients need drainage of extra fluid from different parts of the body?

Extra fluid can accumulate in different body cavities for various reasons. A small amount may not need to be drained, but if the volume is large and affects nearby organs, drainage becomes necessary. Depending on the location, the fluid collection is called by different medical names:

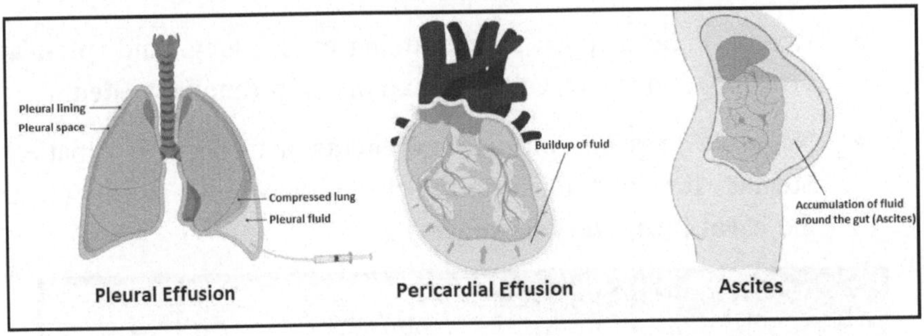

- ➢ **Pleural Effusion**: Fluid around the lungs between two layers of **pleura** (outer lining of lungs). Removal is done via needle or tube—called **pleurocentesis**. If fluid is large, a transparent plastic tube called an **ICD (Intercostal Drain)** is placed between the ribs and connected to a collection bag.
- ➢ **Pericardial Effusion**: Fluid around the heart between the heart muscle and **pericardium** (outer heart covering). If it's large, it may affect heart pumping and lower blood pressure. Doctors remove this by needle or using a **pig-tail catheter** (small tube), and the procedure is called **pericardiocentesis**.

- **Ascites**: Fluid around the intestines in the **abdominal cavity**. Often seen in patients with severe liver disease (**CLD – Chronic Liver Disease**), it causes belly swelling and breathing difficulty. The fluid is drained via needle or catheter through a procedure called **paracentesis** or **ascitic tapping**.
- **Hydrocephalus**: Excess **CSF (Cerebrospinal Fluid** – clear fluid around brain and spinal cord) in the brain. This may cause increased pressure and neurological symptoms. Drainage is done by **lumbar puncture** (needle in the lower back) or by neurosurgical procedures like **EVD (External Ventricular Drain)** or **VP Shunt (Ventriculoperitoneal Shunt)**. With the help of EVD, excessive CSF is collected in a collection bag. But by VP shunt, excessive CSF is drained into body cavity like abdominal cavity where it gets absorbed into the body.

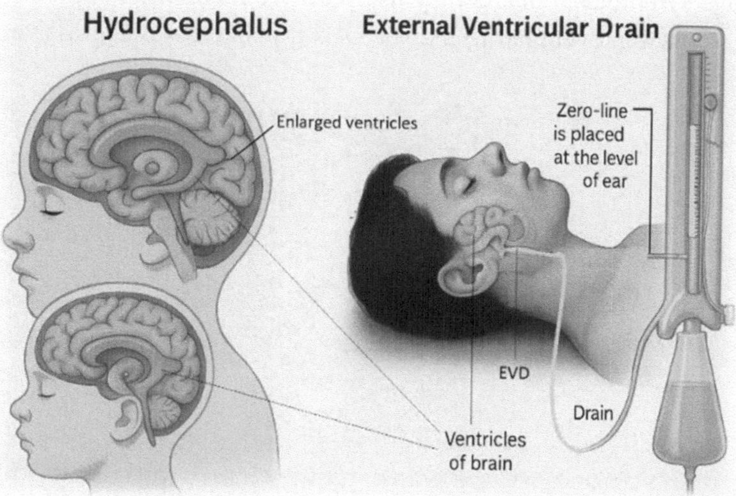

Besides these, patients may require procedures to remove abnormal fluid such as **blood**, **pus**, or **serous fluid** from areas around the liver, kidneys, or bladder:

- **Hematoma**: Collection of blood in one area, usually drained with a **pig-tail catheter**.
- **Abscess**: Collection of pus in organs like liver, spleen, or kidney, also drained using invasive methods.

Q3.23: What is ICU delirium?

Some ICU patients experience sudden behavioural changes during treatment. This is called **ICU delirium**, and it commonly affects elderly and critically ill patients who stay in ICU for more than 24 hours. Symptoms include:

- Confusion
- Hallucinations (seeing or hearing things that aren't real)
- Hyperactivity or reduced alertness
- Disorientation to time, place, or people
- Talking about things that don't make sense or expressing fear of harm

It's difficult for doctors to explain this condition because families may believe everything the patient says due to emotional attachment. To manage symptoms, doctors may use **sedative medicines**, and **restraints** (soft straps to prevent harm) may be used if behaviour is aggressive.

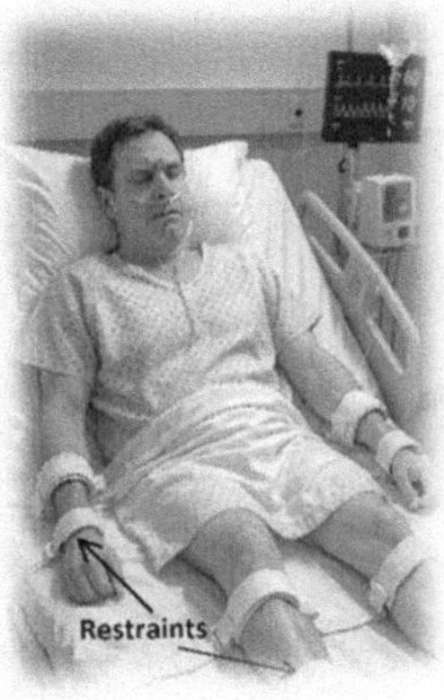

ICU delirium can slow recovery, and symptoms may take days or weeks to resolve. If the patient is not irritable or violent, he or she may be shifted to a regular hospital room. Familiar surroundings and family presence often help reduce delirium symptoms.

Q3.24: What are the risks of blood clots in the ICU, and how are they prevented?

Blood clots are a serious concern in ICU due to **immobility** (lack of movement), which slows blood flow and increases risk of clot formation.

Clots may form in the legs—called **DVT (Deep Vein Thrombosis)**—and may travel to the lungs—called **PE (Pulmonary Embolism)**—which can be life-threatening.

Prevention methods include:

- **Anticoagulation**: Medicines like **heparin** or **enoxaparin** (blood thinner injections) to prevent clot formation.
- **Mechanical Prophylaxis**: Devices like **SCDs (Sequential Compression Devices)** or **TED stockings** (special socks: Thrombo-Embolic Deterrent hose) that improve leg blood flow.
- **Early Mobilization**: Helping patients sit, stand, or walk as soon as medically possible reduces the risk of clots.

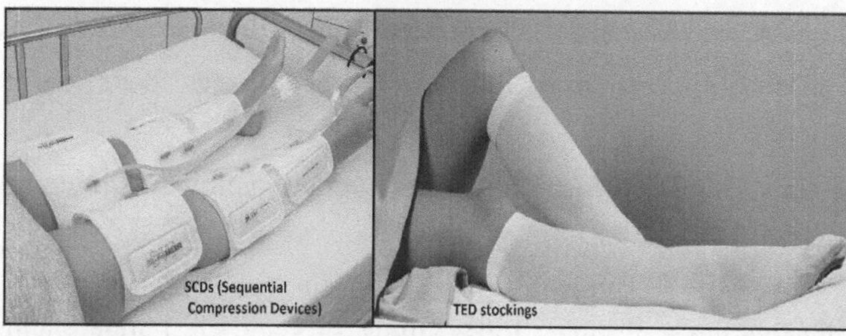

Q3.25: Why do patients develop bed sores if they are bedridden in the ICU for a long time?

Patients in ICU may have limited movement due to illness. Those who lie in bed continuously can develop **pressure sores** or **bed sores** (skin ulcers from prolonged pressure). Constant pressure on skin areas disrupts blood flow. Skin, like any organ, needs **oxygen, glucose**, and **nutrients.** Lack of adequate blood circulation circulation causes skin damage, leading to inflammation and ulcer formation

Patients at higher risk include:

- Those with paralysis
- Elderly or very obese patients unable to walk
- Patients with **spinal, hip**, or **leg fractures**
- Cardiac patients with limited mobility due to breathlessness
- **Intubated patients** on ventilators

- Patients with **critical illness neuropathy** (nerve weakness after ICU stay)
- Patients on **IV infusions** for low blood pressure

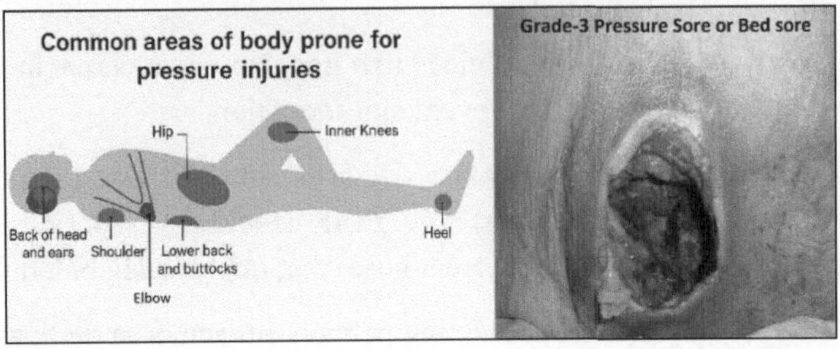

Prevention involves:

- Regularly changing patient's position with back support
- Using **special mattresses** (water beds or air beds) to relieve pressure
- Ensuring good **nutrition**, **skin hygiene**, and maintaining normal blood pressure

Despite all care, pressure sores may still occur due to poor nutrition, low BP, adhesive tapes, frequent loose stools, or swelling. Patients with bed sores may need **daily dressing** of wound and frequent position changes. In some cases, **debridement** (removing dead skin/tissue) or **skin grafting** (surgery to cover wounds) by a **plastic surgeon** may be needed.

Patients may recover from their illness but later face life-threatening **sepsis** (serious infection from bed sores). Families should understand that ICU patients face multiple challenges, and any complication—like a bed sore—can worsen their condition unexpectedly.

Q3.26: What does "shock" and "MODS" (Multiple Organ Dysfunction Syndrome) mean?

Whenever doctors use the word "shock" during counselling about very sick patients, they are referring to extremely low blood pressure. In medical terminology, this is called **profound hypotension** or **shock**.

A patient's blood pressure can drop for several reasons. The most common cause of low blood pressure in the ICU is **sepsis** (a very severe infection that causes high fever, rapid heart rate, and fast breathing). If shock is caused by infection, it is called **septic shock**.

There are other causes of low blood pressure:

- **Hypovolemic shock**: Caused by extreme **dehydration** due to repeated vomiting or diarrhoea.
- **Haemorrhagic shock**: Caused by **significant blood loss**.
- **Cardiogenic shock**: Caused by poor **pumping ability of the heart**.
- **Obstructive shock**: Caused by major **blood clots** in the vessels of the heart or lungs (**pulmonary embolism**).

The function of human organs depends on an uninterrupted and adequate blood supply. When blood pressure is very low for a prolonged period, certain organs begin to malfunction.

- The **kidneys** and **liver** are often affected early. Kidney function tests may show elevated **creatinine levels** (normal value: less than 1.5 mg/dL), and liver function tests may show high levels of liver enzymes.
- Some patients may require **dialysis support** if kidney function worsens quickly due to very low blood pressure.
- If the **brain** is affected, patients may develop symptoms like **confusion** or **altered consciousness**.

To treat such low blood pressure, patients may require:

- **Large volumes of IV fluids** (fluids given through veins)
- **Vasopressor drugs** (medications given by continuous infusion that raise blood pressure)
- **Multiple blood transfusions** in case of haemorrhagic shock
- **Thrombolytic drugs** (clot-busting medicines) in obstructive shock caused by **pulmonary embolism** (sudden blockage in lung blood vessels)
- **Inotropic drugs** (medications that boost heart pumping) in cardiogenic shock caused by heart attacks or heart failure

If blood pressure remains very low despite treatment, few patients may require advanced circulatory support like:

- **ECMO (Extracorporeal Membrane Oxygenation):** A life-support machine that oxygenates blood outside the body. It supports the lungs and heart till the affected organ attains complete recovery.
- **LVAD (Left Ventricular Assist Device):** A mechanical pump that helps the heart pump blood (this device can be considered for the patient who is waiting for heart transplant surgery)

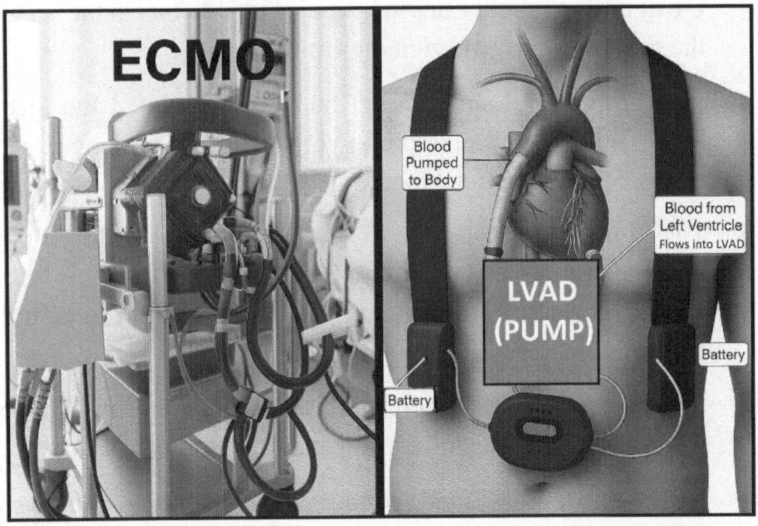

Doctors may use the term **MODS (Multiple Organ Dysfunction Syndrome)** to describe a situation where low blood pressure affects more than two major organs. In MODS, the **heart**, **lungs**, **kidneys**, **liver**, or **brain** may be severely impaired. Once MODS develops, the chances of recovery become lower, and patients are at risk of sudden **cardiac arrest** (cessation of heartbeat) during treatment. Unfortunately, many patients with MODS do not survive, even with intensive care.

Chapter - 4

Different Outcomes and Acceptance

Q4.1: What are some of the most common complications that can occur in the ICU?

Despite the best care, several complications can arise during an ICU stay. It's helpful for families to be aware of these potential issues:

- **Infections**: These include **pneumonia** (lung infection), **bloodstream infections**, and **urinary tract infections (UTIs)**.
- **Delirium**: Sudden confusion and disorientation affecting thinking and behaviour.
- **Blood Clots**: Immobility can increase the risk of clots forming in the legs (**deep vein thrombosis – DVT**) or blood clot traveling to the lungs (**pulmonary embolism – PE**).
- **Skin Breakdown (Pressure Ulcers)**: Bedridden patients are at risk of developing **bedsores** due to continuous pressure on the skin.
- **Muscle Weakness**: Long bed rest and critical illness can reduce muscle strength.
- **Acute Kidney Injury**: The kidneys may be affected by illness or medications, leading to sudden **kidney damage**.
- **Stress Ulcers**: Stress from critical illness may cause ulcers in the **stomach** or **duodenum** (the first part of the small intestine).

Q4.2: What is "CPR"? Why do doctors give CPR to the patient and what are the possible outcomes after CPR?

CPR (Cardio-Pulmonary Resuscitation) is an emergency procedure that helps save a patient's life when the heart has stopped.

- If CPR is performed outside a hospital, it's called **Basic Life Support (BLS)** and can be done by anyone trained.
- In the hospital or ICU, it's called **Advanced Cardiac Life Support (ACLS)**, involving more advanced techniques.

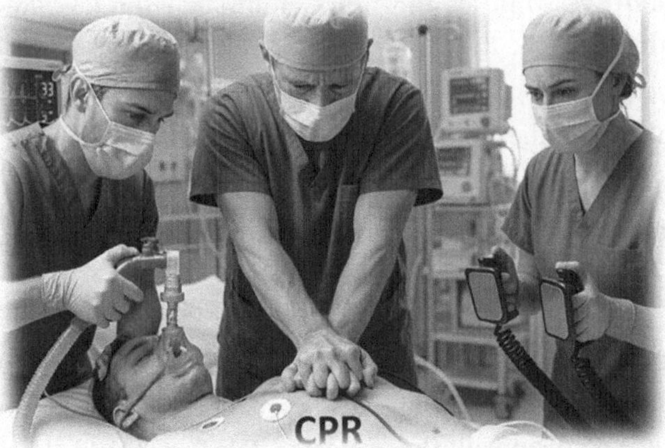

CPR is given when a patient suddenly becomes unconscious and does not have a palpable pulse. It includes **chest compressions** and **breathing support**. In hospital settings, CPR involves:

- **Intubation** (placing a breathing tube through the mouth into the windpipe – trachea)
- Giving **adrenaline injections**
- Using a **DC shock (Direct Current shock)** to correct heart rhythm

If a patient has a pulse—even if unconscious—CPR is **not needed**.

The goal of CPR is to keep blood and oxygen flowing to vital organs while the heart isn't working on its own. If the patient has **arrhythmia** (irregular heart rhythm like very slow or fast rate), the brain may not get enough blood and oxygen, causing unconsciousness. CPR ensures continuous blood supply to the brain until the rhythm is corrected.

Possible outcomes after CPR:

1. **Complete recovery**, if CPR was needed for brief period
2. **Persistent coma-like condition** due to brain damage secondary to poor blood circulation to brain during prolonged CPR
3. **Death**, if the heart doesn't restart despite all efforts

Doctors may be able to revive the heart, but CPR does not treat the underlying disease. Relatives should understand that even after CPR, another cardiac arrest can occur if the underlying health problem isn't resolved.

Q4.3: What is 'therapeutic hypothermia' after CPR, and what are the options for the patient's relatives if the patient remains in a coma?

After **cardiac arrest**, patients in the ICU receive treatment where body temperature is maintained between **34–36°C**. This is called **Therapeutic Hypothermia** or **Targeted Temperature Management**.

- It helps reduce **oxygen demand** by the brain and protects brain cells.
- This cooling treatment is continued for the **first 24 hours**, and patients are given **sedatives** and **muscle relaxants**, so they may not show movements. Breathing support is provided via a **ventilator** (breathing machine).

For the first 24 hours, families should not expect immediate recovery. Doctors may be able to assess **consciousness levels** only after **24 to 36 hours** following CPR.

- If the patient becomes fully alert without brain issues, ventilator support can be taken off within a day or two if there is no major problem with breathing.
- If the patient doesn't regain consciousness even after 36 hours, doctors may suspect **irreversible brain damage** due to lack of oxygen during CPR. This condition is called **Hypoxic Ischemic Encephalopathy**, and it can be confirmed through **MRI of the brain** or **neurological tests** by a specialist. Once confirmed,

families have to decide about further treatment for a comatose patient.

Some families choose to **continue treatment**, in which case they must provide **consent for tracheostomy** (placing a breathing tube through the neck) to continue breathing support for longer duration.

Others may opt for **end-of-life care**, especially if explained clearly about the extent of brain damage and chances of recovery.

Q4.4: What is 'end-of-life care' and 'DNR (Do Not Resuscitate) order' for patients in ICU?

With **advanced age** and **multiple health issues**, many patients arrive at the ICU in a **very critical condition**, and their health may worsen despite appropriate treatment and life support. At a certain stage, doctors may need to inform family members about the **futility of treatment** (no further medical benefit despite the best treatment).

Relatives then have to make decisions about further treatment options when **recovery is unlikely**. These decisions are documented in consent form known as **DNR (Do Not Resuscitate) consent** or **DNAR (Do Not Attempt Resuscitation) consent** or **EOLC (End-of-Life Care) consent.**

These forms include details about the patient's condition and the family's decision to continue or stop certain treatments. They must be signed by the patient's **next of kin** (closest family member).

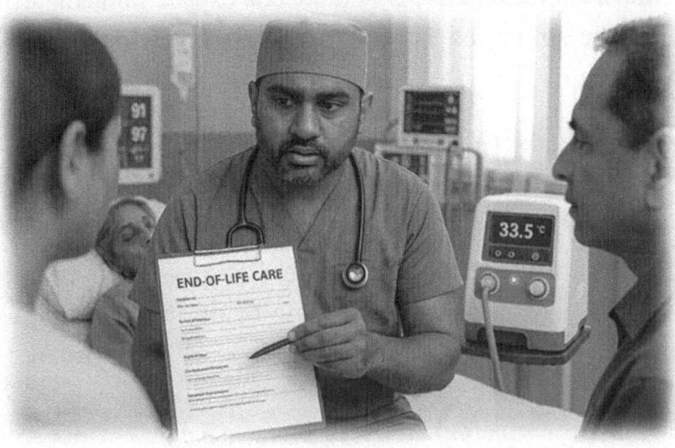

Relatives should understand the difference between:

- **Withholding treatment** (not starting new life-support)
- **Withdrawal of treatment** (stopping existing life-support already in place)

End-of-life care involves continuing basic treatment like medications, nutrition, and comfort care, without starting new **life-sustaining supports** (e.g., ventilator or dialysis) when recovery is highly unlikely.

Usually, **CPR (Cardiopulmonary Resuscitation)** is done when a patient goes into cardiac arrest. But if the patient is already critically ill and receiving multiple supports, CPR may not be beneficial. A signed **DNR consent** helps avoid painful and unnecessary CPR attempts, making it a key part of end-of-life care.

For example, if a critically ill patient is already on **ventilator support** with **low blood pressure**, and doctors recommend **dialysis**, relatives may opt for **non-escalation of treatment** by signing a DNR form.

- If no new life-support is added, it's called **withholding treatment**.
- If current life-support (like ventilator or **vasopressor drugs** [medicines that raise blood pressure]) is stopped, it’s called **withdrawal of treatment**.

Such decisions should be made **jointly** by doctors and relatives when treatment becomes futile. The DNR form is valid only if signed by both parties. Sometimes, relatives may sign the DNR form **early**, even before starting life support.

They can specify which interventions they agree or decline to initiate, such as:

- **Intubation** (placing a breathing tube into the windpipe)
- **NIV support** (Non-Invasive Ventilation using a tight-fitting mask only if patient is conscious)
- **CPR** (Chest compressions and breathing support)
- **Vasopressor support** (continuous medicines to raise blood pressure)

- **Dialysis support**
- **Withdrawal of life support**
- **Withholding treatment**

Choosing end-of-life care can **reduce financial** and **emotional strain** and prevent unnecessary suffering from painful procedures. Ethically, it allows hospitals to use limited resources for other patients with better chances of recovery.

Q4.5: In which clinical scenarios is 'end-of-life care' or a 'DNR order' advisable in the ICU?

People often think **end-of-life care** is only for elderly patients (above 80 years), but even **young patients** may need it if they are critically ill with **multiple organ involvement**.

Common clinical scenarios include:

- Persistent **coma** due to **irreversible brain damage** (from prolonged CPR, brain stroke, bleeding, trauma, or brain infection)
- Continued **shock** (very low blood pressure) with **MODS (Multiple Organ Dysfunction Syndrome)** despite treatment
- Patients with **end-stage liver or kidney disease** not eligible for transplant
- Elderly patients who are **bedridden long-term** with poor quality of life due to conditions like strokes, Parkinson's, or dementia
- Cancer patients with **multiple metastasis** (cancer spread) and poor prognosis
- Elderly patients with **heart failure** and repeated hospital admissions
- Elderly patients with **ILD (Interstitial Lung Disease)** and frequent ICU admissions

Q4.6: What can happen to a patient once 'end-of-life care' is chosen by relatives?

Once **end-of-life care** is opted by patient's relatives, one of the following scenarios may occur:

- Over **90% of patients** with DNR or end-of-life consent will experience **further deterioration** and eventually go into **cardiac arrest**. Relatives should understand that **death is expected**, and it may occur within **hours or days**.
- If the patient is on **ventilator support** with **high vasopressor doses**, death can occur within minutes or hours once support is withdrawn.
- A few patients may remain clinically stable with only supportive care—not worsening or improving. Such patients can be shifted to a ward, private room, or rehabilitation centre. They do not need to stay in the ICU.
- Occasionally, few patients with prior signed DNR consent may improve gradually during ICU stay. Some of them may recover enough to be discharged home.

Hence, DNR or end-of-life care does not always mean "end of life." It simply informs doctors that the patient's relatives do not want **aggressive treatments** (CPR, dialysis, intubation, vasopressors) if the patient's condition worsens.

Q4.7: How is the decision made to withdraw or withhold life-sustaining treatment?

The decision to **withdraw or withhold treatment** is complex. It is made through discussion between:

- The **medical team**
- The **patient,** if capable
- The **family members**

Key factors considered include:

- The patient's **current medical condition and likely outcome**
- The patient's **wishes** (based on advance directives or past conversations)
- The **balance of burdens** versus **benefits** from further treatment
- **Ethical** and **legal considerations**

The goal is to make a decision that aligns with the patient's **best interest** and **personal values.**

Q4.8: What is palliative care, and how can it help in the ICU?

Palliative care is specialized medical support for patients with **serious illness**, aimed at relieving **symptoms** and **stress**. Its goal is to improve **quality of life** for both the patient and family.

In the ICU, palliative care can help by:

- Managing pain and discomfort
- Addressing emotional and spiritual concerns
- Assisting with difficult decisions
- Providing support to family members

Palliative care can be **given alongside curative treatments**, and is **not the same as hospice care**, which is typically reserved for terminally ill patients.

Q4.9: What is the death declaration process in the ICU?

Different hospitals may have their own protocols for declaring death in the ICU. Every doctor has a different approach to communicating with the patient's relatives during such sensitive moments.

Breaking bad news is emotionally challenging for doctors, and relatives should understand that patients may succumb due to their underlying **medical condition**. No health professional is responsible for a patient's death if it results from the disease itself. Not all medical conditions are curable, and some patients may deteriorate despite proper treatment in the ICU.

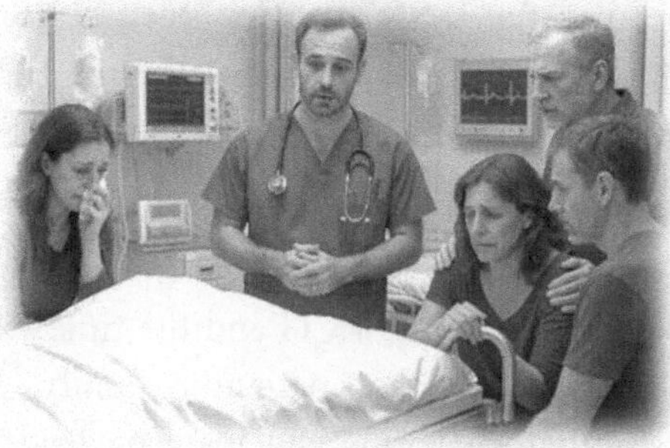

In many cases, doctors must inform the family about the **poor prognosis** (very low chance of recovery), especially when a critically ill patient may experience **cardiac arrest** (sudden stopping of the heart) at any time. For most ICU deaths, the patient's condition worsens gradually during treatment. Doctors can then counsel and prepare the family for possible outcomes, including death.

However, **sudden cardiac arrest** can also occur in stable patients who are getting treated in wards or rooms.

Common causes for sudden cardiac arrest include:

- **Massive heart attack**
- **Arrhythmias** (abnormal heart rhythms)
- **Pulmonary embolism** (blood clot in lung vessels)
- **Intracranial bleed** (bleeding in the brain)
- **Rupture of major blood vessels**

When a patient suffers cardiac arrest in the ICU, **CPR (cardiopulmonary resuscitation)** is started immediately by doctors. A member from ICU team may inform the relatives immediately so they can be present near the ICU. Sometimes, one doctor performs CPR while another speaks with the family. Once CPR is completed, doctors discuss the outcome.

If the patient does not respond even after prolonged CPR (around 20 minutes), doctors document a **flat-line ECG** (electrocardiogram with no heart activity) to confirm death. The time noted on this ECG is considered the **exact time of death** and is recorded on the **death certificate**.

If cardiac arrest occurs after **DNR (Do Not Resuscitate) order** is signed by patient's family members, doctors may take the ECG without doing CPR. The flat-line ECG also serves to document the time of death.

Sometimes, doctors may be attending to other ICU emergencies, so they may not inform relatives immediately. This can cause a **mismatch** between the time recorded on the ECG and the time when the family is notified. In such circumstances, patient's family members should understand that simultaneous emergencies can lead to delay in the declaration of death.

Once death is declared:

- Nursing staff can remove all the tubes, lines, and devices from the patient.
- If the **ventilator** is still connected, relatives may see slight chest movements. This is due to machine pressure and not actual breathing.
- Doctors may allow relatives to spend a few minutes near the patient after the death declaration.
- The body is then covered and handed over after completing all documentation.

If relatives wish, they can request:

- Specific clothes to be placed on patient's body
- Hospital sheets or their own cloth to cover the body
- **Mortuary freezer box** (mostly outsourced) if they need to preserve the body for a few days

This may be needed if they are waiting for some close relatives to arrive from remote place or if they want to transport the body to a distant location. Not all hospitals have **mortuary freezer** facilities, but hospital staff can help locate nearby providers.

Chapter - 5

What Happens After the ICU?

Q5.1: What is a step-down unit?

A **step-down unit** is a transitional area for patients who are **stable** but still need **close monitoring** before moving to a general ward or going home. Since patients in the step-down unit are more stable, one nurse can attend 2–3 patients.

Intensivists (critical care doctors) or other physicians perform **daily assessments** to monitor progress. Patients are moved to general wards or rooms from the step-down unit once they are almost fully recovered.

Q5.2: Why do patients need to be shifted to rooms or wards from the ICU?

Sometimes, patient's relatives request a direct discharge from the ICU, but doctors may recommend shifting the patient to a room or ward first. When patients are recovering, it's better to observe them in a less intensive setting to confirm they are fit for discharge.

If no new medical issues occur in the room or ward, it's more likely the patient will remain stable after going home. Some patients take longer time to recover from critical illness and they have to stay in the ICU for an extended period. Once they become **hemodynamically stable** (normal blood pressure and heart rate), they can be moved to a room or ward. Doctors always insist to shift the patients to room or wards because prolonged ICU exposure increases the risk of **infections**.

If they no longer need ICU machines or equipment, continuous observation can be done outside the ICU. After major surgeries, patients often need nursing support for a few days. By keeping them in a room or ward before discharge, family can monitor patient's requirements during the transition from full support to minimal assistance. This provides extra confidence to both patient and family that there are no unexpected post-surgery problems.

Q5.3: What is ICU rehabilitation, and why do some patients need to stay in a rehabilitation centre before going home?

Rehabilitation is the process that helps patients recover from illness or injury and regain their physical and mental strength.

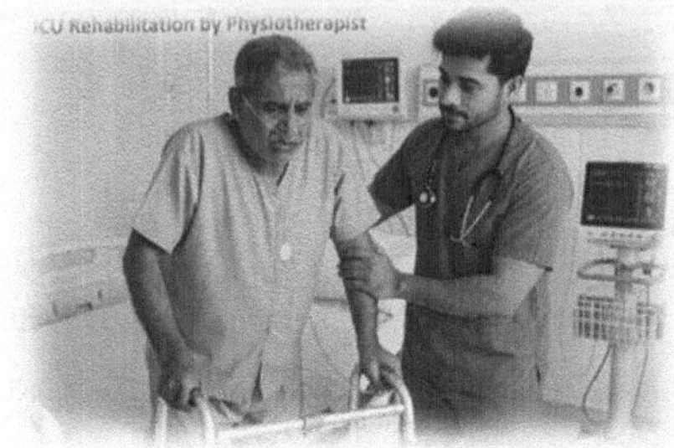

Leaving the ICU does not mean that the ICU journey is over—it begins a **new phase** of rebuilding strength, function, and well-being. Some patients may experience **physical and emotional setbacks** even after surviving a critical illness.

Patients are assessed by a **multidisciplinary team** including intensivists, physicians, nurses, nutritionists, physiotherapists, and respiratory therapists.

This team evaluates the patient's **specific limitations** and creates a **personalized treatment plan**.

- **Physiotherapy** plays a crucial role in rebuilding **strength and mobility**.
- Due to prolonged bed rest, many patients develop **muscle weakness** or **atrophy** (loss of muscle mass).
- Therapists guide patients through exercises—from simple movements to walking and climbing stairs.
- **Respiratory therapy** is important for patients who were on **ventilator support**, especially for pneumonia.

Respiratory therapists teach the patients **breathing exercises** and how to use devices like the **incentive spirometer** (a clear tool with coloured balls or piston that moves during breathing to train the lungs). These therapies begin in the ICU and continue afterward.

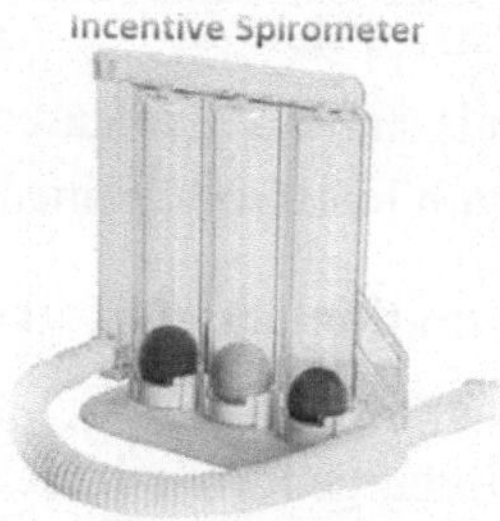

If the hospital doesn't have a dedicated rehabilitation facility, doctors may recommend transferring the patient to a **rehabilitation centre** after ICU discharge. Patient's stay at rehabilitation centre is very important because there are less chances of **hospital-acquired infections** during the long-term recovery.

Q5.4: What happens when my loved one is ready to leave the ICU?

Leaving the ICU means your loved one has made **significant progress** and is stable enough for a lower level of care.

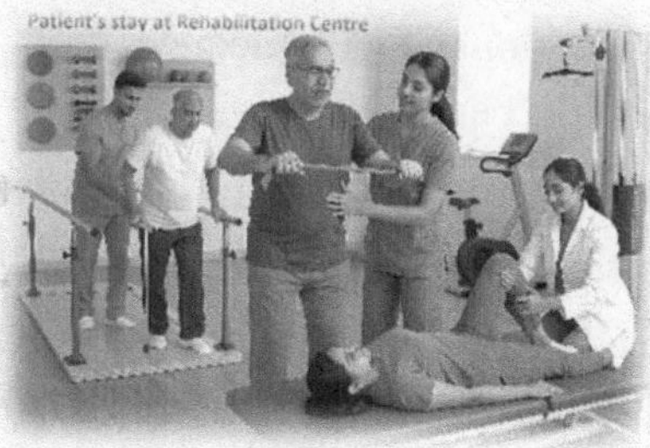

There are **four possible places** they may be transferred to:

1. General Ward or Private Room

If no longer needing **oxygen support** or **constant monitoring**, the patient can be shifted there.

2. Step-Down Unit

This unit offers care that is less intensive than the ICU but more advanced than a ward. It's for patients who still need **oxygen therapy** or occasional monitoring.

3. Rehabilitation Centre

If your loved one requires **intensive rehabilitation** (e.g., after a major stroke), they may be transferred to a rehabilitation facility.

4. Home (with nursing care at home)

In some cases, if the patient is stable and requires only **basic nursing care**, they can recover at home with help from trained caregivers or nurses.

Q5.5: What kind of information should I gather from the ICU team before discharge?

Before your loved one is discharged from the ICU, it's important to collect detailed information from the medical team to ensure safe recovery at home:

- **Diagnosis and Medical History**: Ask for a written summary describing the illness, ICU treatments, and relevant past conditions.
- **Medications**: Request a list of all medicines—names, doses, timing, and how they should be taken (by mouth, injection, etc.).
- **Follow-Up Appointments**: Confirm any scheduled visits with specialists or general physicians.
- **Dietary Instructions**: Get guidance on what your loved one should or shouldn't eat.
- **Activity Restrictions**: Ask about any physical limitations (like avoiding stairs, lifting, or walking long distances).
- **Wound Care Instructions**: If applicable, learn how to clean and dress wounds properly.
- **Equipment Needs**: Check if devices like a **wheelchair, walker, oxygen cylinder, portable CPAP/Bi-PAP machine** or **feeding tube** are needed.
- **Emergency Contact Information**: Make sure you have updated phone numbers for doctors and emergency services.
- **Rehabilitation Plan**: Understand the schedule and goals for continued recovery through physiotherapy or other therapies.

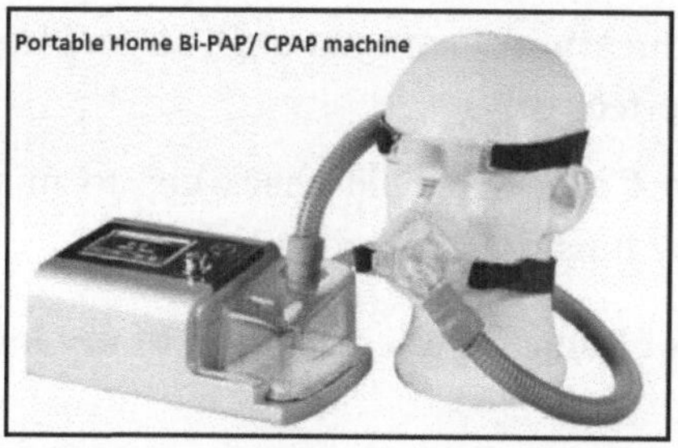

Q5.6: What is "Post-Intensive Care Syndrome (PICS)"?

Post-Intensive Care Syndrome (PICS) is a condition that affects both patients and their families after a prolonged ICU stay.

For **patients**, symptoms may include:

- Extreme fatigue
- Memory loss
- Trouble focusing
- Anxiety or depression

For **families**, symptoms may appear as:

- Constant worry about the patient
- Nightmares or flashbacks from the ICU experience
- Feeling of helplessness or burnout

Q5.7: How can "Post-Intensive Care Syndrome (PICS)" be prevented and managed?

Preventing and managing PICS involves multiple strategies:

- **Early Mobilization**: Encourage the patient to sit up, move, or walk as soon as they are stable.
- **Pain Management**: Ensure the patient receives proper pain relief.
- **Cognitive Stimulation**: Engage in activities that challenge memory and thinking, like reading, puzzles, or conversation.
- **Mental Health Support**: Provide access to counsellors or therapists for emotional care.
- **Rehabilitation Services**: Arrange physical, occupational, or speech therapy as needed.

- **Family Education**: Learn about PICS and how to care for your loved one effectively.
- **Follow-Up Care**: Schedule check-ups to monitor recovery and manage any lingering symptoms.

Q5.8: What kind of home care services might my loved one need after discharge?

Home care should be arranged based on the patient's condition. Here are common services to consider:

➢ **Nursing Care**: If the patient needs:

- IV medications
- Feeding tube support
- Wound dressing changes
- Urinary catheter care

You'll need to arrange a trained nurse for home visits.

➢ **Physiotherapy**: Ongoing physical exercises—either active (performed by the patient) or passive (assisted)—are essential for recovery.

A physiotherapist should guide and monitor these activities to rebuild strength and mobility.

➢ **Oxygen Therapy**: If the patient still requires oxygen after recovery from conditions like **pneumonia**, arrange for:

- Oxygen cylinders
- Oxygen concentrators

Such equipment must be available at home before discharge.

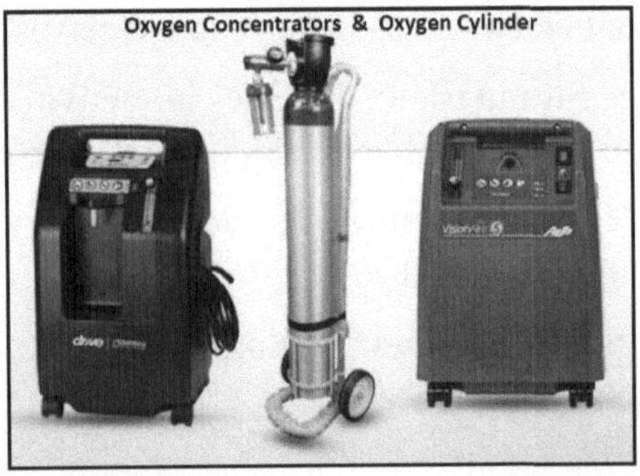

Chapter - 6

Most Common Medical Conditions for Which Patient Needs ICU Stay!

It is very difficult for patient's relatives to understand complex medical terminology used for the patient's clinical problem. Once the basic reason behind patient's ailment is identified, doctors generally explain it clearly by providing exact diagnosis. [**Diagnosis** means identification of disease, condition or injury] There might be hundreds of medical problems for which patients may need treatment in ICU but there are few most encountered diagnoses in ICU which can be the major reason for the admission in ICU. Patient's relatives can ask the doctors about "provisional diagnosis" once the basic investigations are done. [**Provisional diagnosis** means a tentative diagnosis made by doctors when they suspect a particular condition but need more information to be certain]

It is practically impossible for patients and their families to learn everything about all diseases. However, once a diagnosis is established by doctors, they often begin to have multiple questions about that specific condition. If they possess basic knowledge about the disease, the necessary investigations required for diagnosis, and the available treatment options, they are less likely to experience anxiety or confusion during the counselling session—because they already have some understanding of the diagnosis. This enables them to ask relevant questions to ICU doctors during the counselling session. Here is a small list of common diagnosis (medical condition) with which patients get admitted to ICU.

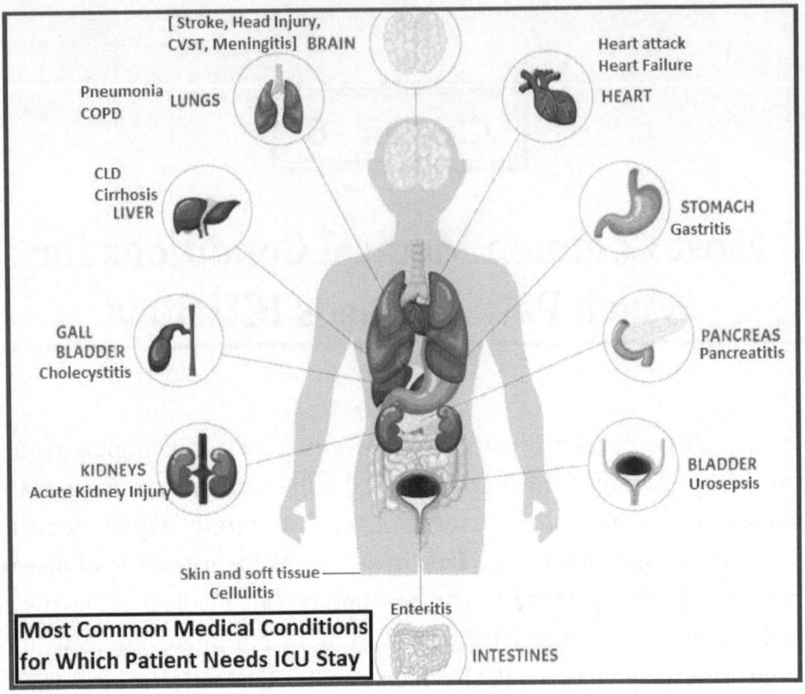

Brain:

- Stroke
- Head injury with intracranial brain haemorrhage
- CVT or CVST [cerebral venous thrombosis or cerebral venous sinus thrombosis]
- Meningitis

Lungs:

- Pneumonia
- COPD [Chronic Obstructive Pulmonary disease]

Heart:

- Heart attack [myocardial infarction]
- Heart failure

Liver:

- CLD [Chronic liver disease] and Liver Cirrhosis

Pancreas:

- Pancreatitis

Gall bladder:

- Cholecystitis

Kidneys and Urinary bladder:

- Urosepsis with acute kidney injury

Skin and soft tissues:

- Cellulitis

Intestines:

- Gastroenteritis

Diagnosis: 6.1 Stroke

It is a medical emergency in which the patient may develop sudden neurological symptoms, which may include weakness in the leg or arm, slurring of speech, giddiness, inability to walk properly, inability to hold things, headache, or altered conscious level.

There are two main types of brain stroke:

a. Ischemic Stroke (blockage in blood vessels of the brain)

b. Haemorrhagic Stroke (bleeding in the brain)

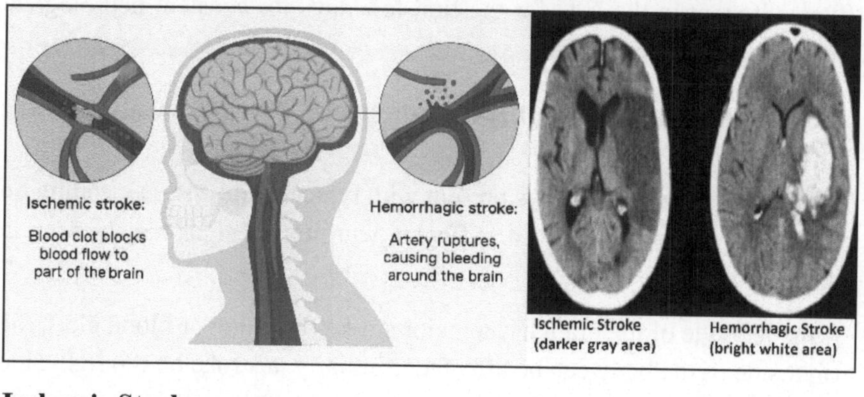

Ischemic Stroke:

This type of stroke occurs when blood does not reach a particular part of the brain due to a blood clot in one of the brain's vessels (**blood vessels** are tubes through which blood flows to organs).

Haemorrhagic Stroke:

This type of stroke occurs when blood leaks into a part of the brain, usually because of the sudden rupture of a blood vessel due to extremely high blood pressure (in that case, such type of stroke is known as **hypertensive bleed**) or abnormal vessel structure (if abnormal dilated blood vessel get ruptured, it is called **aneurysmal bleed**).

The treatment strategy is different for each type of stroke. For ischemic stroke, blood thinner drugs are started for the patient, and if the patient presents with haemorrhagic stroke, blood thinner drugs should be avoided. The reason for bleeding in the brain must be identified first, and treatment is continued accordingly.

Any part of the body can swell once it is injured. Similarly, the area of the brain affected by stroke can also swell in the first 3–4 days after the onset. Such swelling can increase pressure inside the brain. Since the brain is surrounded by the bony skull, there is no extra space for brain to expand, which can lead to excessive intracranial (inside the skull) pressure and further compression of vital brain structures.

To prevent this, doctors may start **hyperosmolar therapy** (injections like 3% saline and mannitol) to reduce the brain pressure if swelling is suspected or anticipated. This treatment is common for both types of strokes and must be continued in the ICU, which is why stroke patients are typically kept in the ICU for the first few days for constant neurological monitoring.

Q6.1.1: Why do some patients with stroke develop paralysis while others do not?

Brain stroke does not always present with typical paralysis. Depending on the area of the brain involved, different neurological signs may be seen in different patients.

If the left side of the brain has a major stroke (bleeding or blood clot), the right side of the body can be affected. Similarly, a stroke on the right side of the brain can cause weakness on the left side of the body.

If the stroke affects certain areas, there may not be any weakness on either side, but other signs like giddiness or difficulty in swallowing. These occur when the **cerebellum** (part of brain which is responsible for balance and coordination) or **midbrain** (central brain area involved in swallowing, coughing, and breathing) are affected.

Sometimes, stroke may affect only a small area of the brain (**lacunar infarct**: a tiny part affected by ischemic stroke); such strokes may not cause obvious weakness, although MRI (Magnetic Resonance Imaging) of the brain may still show changes.

Rarely, few patients may show stroke-like symptoms for just a few minutes and return to normal quickly. This is called a **TIA (Transient Ischemic Attack)** and requires further tests like MRI of the brain.

Q6.1.2: Why is time very crucial in treating stroke patients?

If the patient arrives at the hospital within 4.5 hours of symptom onset, they may be offered **thrombolysis** (an injection that dissolves blood clots) in cases of ischemic stroke (not haemorrhagic stroke).

Thrombolysis involves breaking down the clot using specialized drugs like **Alteplase** or **Tenecteplase**, administered after ruling out any evidence of bleeding in the brain with the help of CT scan or MRI of the brain.

Before giving this injection, the doctor explains the major side effect: **bleeding**, which can occur anywhere, including the brain. Since the benefits usually outweigh the risks, relatives often give consent to this treatment. Some patients improve within 24 hours, while others may worsen due to bleeding into the area of the initial stroke. Doctors may use the word "**haemorrhagic conversion**" if bleeding happens inside the ischemic stroke area.

If the patient with ischemic stroke arrives late (after 4.5 hours), patient is treated with **antiplatelet drugs** (blood thinners) and **statins** (to reduce cholesterol levels) in case of ischemic stroke.

A few patients with major vessel blockage may be eligible for **mechanical thrombectomy** (a catheter-based procedure done in a Cath-lab by a neuro-intervention specialist to remove the blood clot from affected blood vessel of the brain).

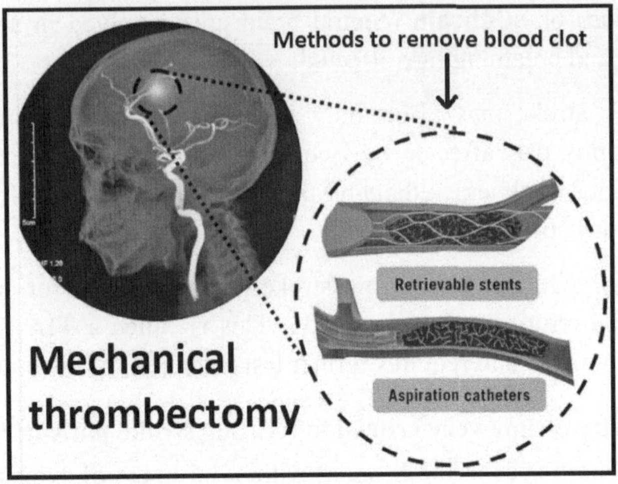

Q6.1.3: How long does it take to recover from a stroke?

Recovery from stroke depends on multiple factors like patient's age, comorbid conditions (long term health issues like high blood pressure and diabetes), area of brain involved, size of stroke and time of presentation to the hospital after the onset of stroke symptoms.

- If thrombolysis restores blood flow effectively, some patients may improve within 24 hours. Others may take a few days, even after thrombolysis. Doctors may request a repeat CT scan of the brain 24 hours after thrombolysis to check for bleeding.
- Most stroke patients take weeks to months for full recovery, depending on stroke severity and brain area affected.
- Some may recover only partially after 6 months and need help in walking. Others may not recover at all and remain bedridden.
- For faster recovery, stroke patients need regular **physiotherapy**, and some may need to stay in a **rehabilitation centre** for a few weeks after discharge.

Q6.1.4: Why do some patients deteriorate a few days after stroke, despite ongoing treatment?

Not all stroke patients have the same outcomes. Some improve quickly, while others worsen—even with appropriate treatment.

In the first few days, swelling around the stroke area may increase pressure in the brain tissue. Since the brain is enclosed in the skull with no room to expand, this increased pressure [also known as **raised ICP (Intracranial Pressure)**] can compress vital areas and cause coma.

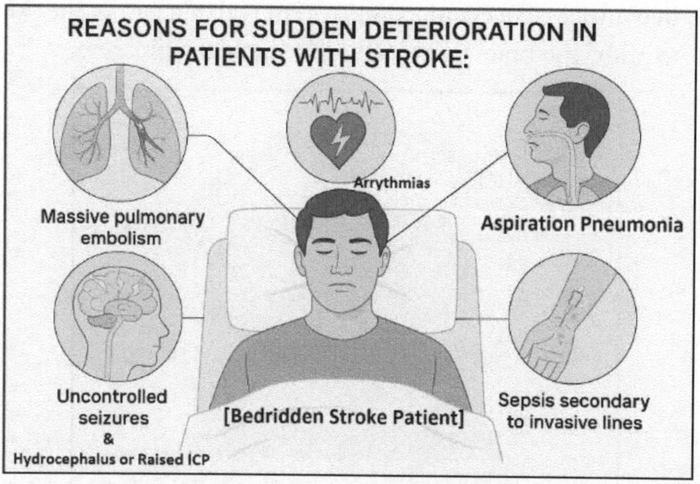

There are few more other reasons for sudden deterioration in patients with stroke:

- Infections like **aspiration pneumonia** (it occurs in patients who are semiconscious or unconscious because pneumonia may occur easily if aspiration is happening due to entry of saliva, secretions or stomach content into lungs), **ventilator-associated pneumonia** (type of pneumonia which can occur in few patients after 2 days of invasive ventilator support), **bedsores**, or **catheter-related infections** (infections associated with indwelling catheters and tubes like central line or urine catheter)
- Uncontrolled **seizures** (fits)
- **Hydrocephalus** (accumulation of cerebrospinal fluid in the brain)
- **Cardiac arrhythmias** (abnormal heart rhythms)
- **Massive pulmonary embolism** (obstructed blood flow to the lungs due to big blood clot formation in blood vessels carrying blood to lungs), often arising from **DVT – Deep Vein Thrombosis** (blood clot in leg veins due to poor mobility)

Q6.1.5: What surgeries may be needed for stroke patients?

- Not all stroke patients require surgery. However, if **intracranial pressure** (pressure inside of skull) becomes dangerously high, neurosurgeons may recommend a procedure called **decompressive craniectomy**—removal of a part of the skull bone to allow the brain to expand and relieve the pressure.

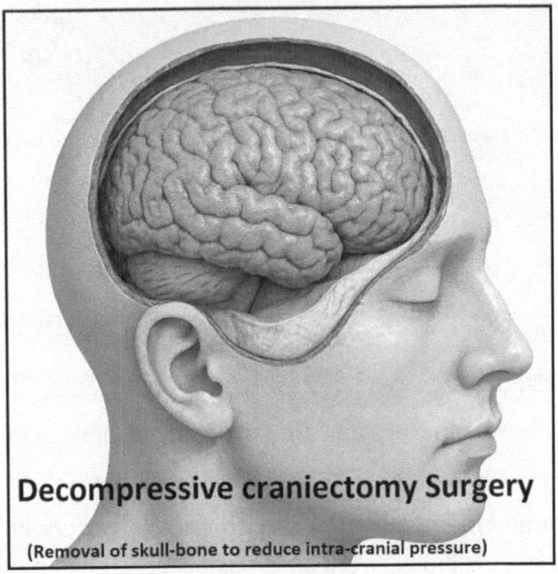

- Patient's relatives should understand that the decompressive craniectomy surgery does not reverse brain damage but helps to prevent further damage. It is considered a life-saving emergency procedure.

- The removed skull piece is preserved—either in a freezer or under the skull of the abdomen (subcutaneous pocket)—until the patient recovers.

- After complete recovery through rehabilitation and physiotherapy, the patient may undergo **cranioplasty** (surgery to reattach the bone and repair the skull defect).

Q6.1.6: Why do patients remain comatose despite neurosurgery after a major stroke?

Sometimes, neurological damage can be very extensive due to a major brain stroke, despite adequate attempts to reduce excessive pressure in the brain. Many patients with stroke need emergency craniectomy as a life-saving intervention and can be saved by such surgery, but sometimes their conscious level does not improve even after surgery.

This can happen due to excessive brain damage secondary to low blood supply and low oxygen delivery to a specific part of the brain. Such patients may develop **"hypoxic brain damage"** (irreversible brain damage due to low oxygen reaching the brain) and may remain comatose despite emergency neurosurgical intervention. A post-operative CT scan of the brain can help to understand the damage caused by extensive pressure in the brain.

A few patients may show improvement very slowly (weeks to months) after emergency craniectomy and may require prolonged ventilator support and intensive care.

Q6.1.7: Why do doctors advise intubation and ventilator support even if the patient is conscious and breathing normally?

Whenever doctors inform about the need for intubation and ventilator support, the patient's relatives often assume the patient is extremely critical and may not recover once ventilator support is initiated. Due to such concerns, some relatives hesitate to sign consent for intubation and mechanical ventilation.

Patient's relatives should first understand the exact reason for intubation. Some stroke patients may gradually lose consciousness and have a high chance of aspiration (entry of food particles, saliva, or secretions into the breathing pipe). Hence, ventilator support becomes mandatory for airway protection.

Some stroke patients may develop involvement of **bulbar muscles** (muscles in the mouth and throat that control speech and swallowing), leading to excessive retention of saliva that cannot be swallowed properly. Such patients start coughing immediately after drinking even a sip of water, or their oxygen saturation may drop gradually if aspiration (entry of saliva, secretions or stomach content into lungs) continues. This can eventually lead to aspiration pneumonia, which may delay recovery or, in some cases, become life-threatening.

Patient's relatives should understand that even conscious patients without initial breathing issues may still have swallowing difficulties due to the stroke's specific location. To prevent further aspiration, intubation is compulsory in such cases.

Q6.1.8: Why do stroke patients sometimes need tracheostomy?

Not all stroke patients require ventilator support, and not all patients on ventilators require **tracheostomy** (placing a breathing tube through the neck directly into the windpipe). Relatives should understand that tracheostomy helps prevent aspiration—once the tracheostomy tube is in place, food particles or secretions cannot enter the trachea, making airway protection the main reason for tracheostomy in stroke patients.

If patients begin to recover within 4 to 5 days of ventilator support, tracheostomy is not needed. Doctors first attempt to remove ventilator support, but if the patient requires **re-intubation** (inserting the breathing tube again if patient doesn't breathe adequately after removal of ventilator support) within a day, tracheostomy is the ideal choice.

If a patient remains unconscious or semi-conscious after 4–5 days of treatment, ventilator support cannot be removed until the patient becomes alert and coherent. Such patients need tracheostomy, and ventilator support may continue for a prolonged period through the tracheostomy.

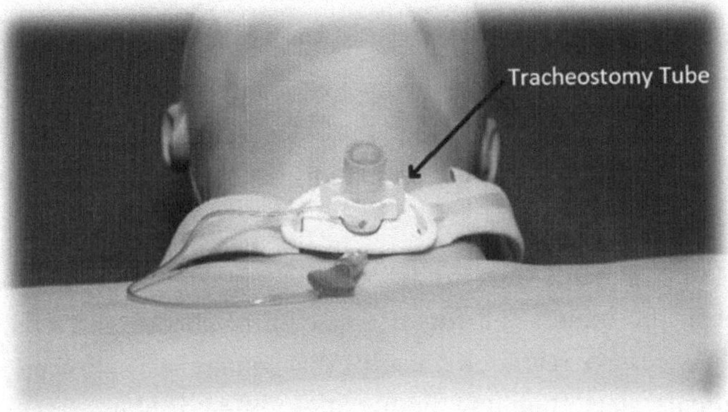

If a patient is on ventilator support solely due to bulbar muscle weakness (difficulty swallowing and clearing oral secretions), tracheostomy is necessary for a longer duration, as recovery from such strokes can take weeks.

Q6.1.9: How long must patients be fed through a feeding tube after a major stroke? Is there an alternative?

Some stroke patients have difficulty swallowing and may require a feeding tube to receive liquid supplements and diet. This is called a "**Ryle's tube**," placed through the nostril to bypass the mouth, throat, and oesophagus (food-pipe) and deliver food directly into the stomach. Once the patient can swallow liquids without coughing, the tube is removed, and regular oral feeding is resumed.

Patients with tracheostomy also receive food through a Ryle's tube if the breathing tube is in place. After full recovery, the tracheostomy tube is removed (a process called "**decannulation**"), and the Ryle's tube can also be removed. The patient can then start oral intake.

If the patient is semi-conscious and severely affected, recovery may take months. In such cases, doctors advise switching to a **PEG tube (Percutaneous Endoscopic Gastrostomy)**.

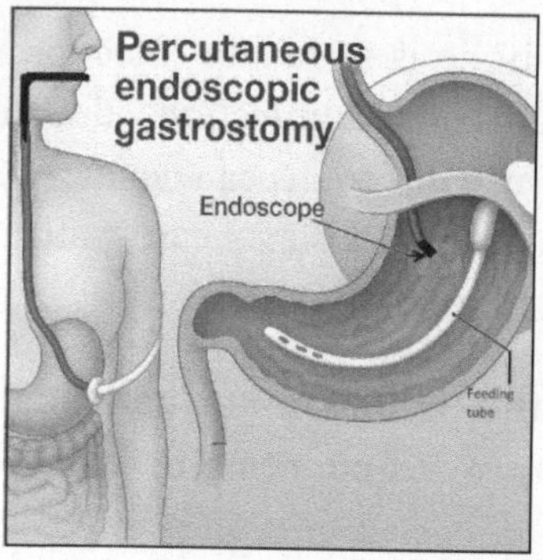

This PEG tube, placed by a medical gastroenterologist using an endoscope, enters the stomach through the skin of the abdomen. It's wider than a Ryle's tube and can remain for months. Home-prepared crushed or liquid food can be given through this tube. Relatives must learn how to feed through a PEG tube and remember to flush it with water after each feeding to keep it clean and functional.

Q6.1.10: Why do doctors insist on shifting stroke patients to rehabilitation centres?

It's important to understand the difference between a hospital and a rehabilitation centre. Hospitals have ICUs for very sick patients, whereas rehabilitation centres do not admit critically ill individuals. Once patients start recovering from stroke or serious illness, they need regular physiotherapy and mobilization.

Although physiotherapy is available in ICU, frequent and intensive sessions are difficult to manage in that setting. A dedicated rehabilitation centre offers structured therapy to accelerate recovery, making it the best option after ICU discharge if full recovery hasn't yet occurred.

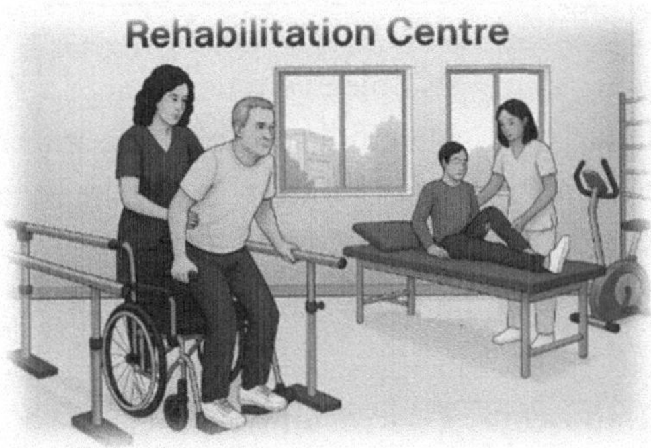

Another reason for shifting is to reduce infection risk. ICU patients are vulnerable to hospital-acquired infections due to proximity to other critically ill patients. Such infections can delay recovery. Therefore, once stable and no longer needing ICU-level care, patients should be shifted to a rehabilitation centre for continued recovery.

Q6.1.11: What are the options for a patient's relatives if a stroke patient does not improve and remains comatose for a prolonged duration?

Not all stroke patients recover fully. Some improve slowly over months; others may show signs of recovery within weeks. Many may remain unconscious or semi-conscious for a long time.

Some stroke patients breathe independently but remain in a coma permanently. They usually breathe through a tracheostomy tube and are fed through a feeding tube.

At times, relatives may find it financially or emotionally difficult to continue prolonged ICU treatment. These are the main reasons behind decisions to withhold or withdraw treatment.

If chances of recovery are less and the patient remains unconscious or comatose, relatives can consider the following options:

a. **Rehabilitation centre** care, if the patient breathes adequately without ventilator support

b. **End-of-life care**, if the patient is comatose and dependent on a ventilator—relatives may sign consent to withdraw ventilator and other supportive treatment (without which the patient may pass away)

c. **Home care**, if the patient has a tracheostomy and requires nutritional support via a Ryle's tube (feeding tube)—relatives can arrange for nursing support at home.

Diagnosis: 6.2 Head Injury with Brain Haemorrhage

Road traffic accidents, falls from height, or a direct hit by a heavy object can cause serious head injury, which may lead to bleeding inside the brain [**ICH: Intracranial Haemorrhage**]. Depending on the area of the brain where bleeding occurs, doctors may use different terminology for such bleeding:

1. **SDH** – Subdural Hematoma (blood collection under the outer layer of the brain)

2. **EDH** – Extradural Hematoma (blood collection outside the outer layer of the brain)

3. **SAH** – Subarachnoid Haemorrhage (diffuse bleeding in multiple areas of the brain)

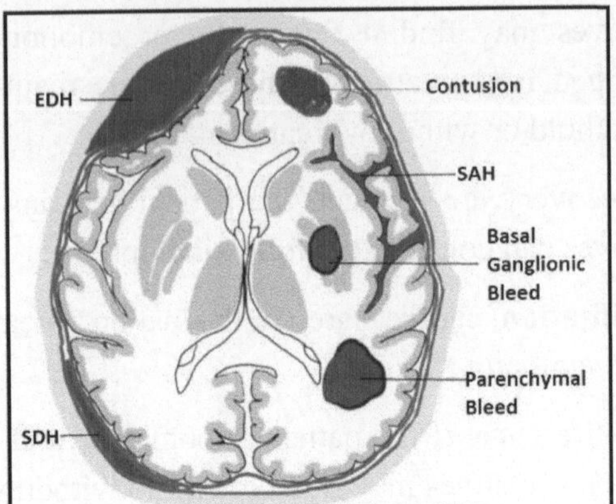

Types of Brain Haemorrhage

Sometimes, head injury causes bruising in brain tissue, known as a **contusion**. Minor contusions may heal within a couple of days with rest and medication. Since the brain is enclosed in a tight bony skull, there is no space for blood to escape, and swelling or bleeding can lead to a dangerous increase in pressure inside the skull. Many patients may die immediately after a serious head injury if such **intracranial pressure** rises abruptly to the extent that vital brain structures become compressed, and the patient may succumb within seconds to minutes.

Q6.2.1: Why do some patients show irritable and aggressive behaviour in the ICU after head injury?

Whenever the brain is affected by injury, bleeding, or stroke, the brain tissue undergoes changes. Brain cells may swell, and brain coverings can become irritated. These organic changes cause behavioural and neurological symptoms.

Many patients admitted to the ICU after head injury exhibit extremely violent, non-cooperative behaviour and irrelevant speech, especially if they have contusions or bleeding. Such patients may need **physical restraints** (tying hands and legs to the ICU bed) and **sedative drugs** (medications that calm aggression and induce sleep), which act as **chemical restraints**.

With **hyperosmolar therapy** (medications which can reduce brain pressure) and supportive care, some patients begin improving within a few days, and their behaviour returns to normal. Until then, ICU monitoring is necessary.

Q6.2.2: Why does the patient need a repeat CT scan of the brain after head injury, even if their condition remains unchanged in the ICU?

Once the brain is injured and bleeding occurs, swelling of brain is inevitable. Though the patient may be receiving treatment to reduce brain pressure, early signs of worsening may be seen by comparing new CT images with previous ones. If the new scan shows increased bleeding and compression of adjacent brain structures, **emergency surgery** may be needed.

A patient may deteriorate suddenly due to an abrupt pressure increase. If surgery is delayed, the chances of recovery decrease. To prevent this, doctors repeat CT scans frequently during the first 3–4 days post-injury to detect major changes early and guide neurosurgical decisions.

Relatives should feel reassured if subsequent CT scans do not show worsening. They should understand that doctors never advise unnecessary tests. Even normal results are useful to rule out worsening. Some tests are mandatory to detect problems early, so repeat scans should not be a concern.

Q6.2.3: What type of neurosurgery may be needed in case of brain haemorrhage?

Based on the type and location of the brain injury, neurosurgeons may recommend:

- **Burr Hole Surgery** – drilling small holes in the skull to relieve pressure
- **EVD Surgery (External Ventricular Drain)** – placing a tube inside the brain to drain the fluid (CSF-cerebrospinal Fluid)
- **DECRA Surgery (Decompressive Craniectomy)** – removing a part of the skull bone to allow brain swelling. Opening the skull to access brain tissue is considered as **Craniotomy**.

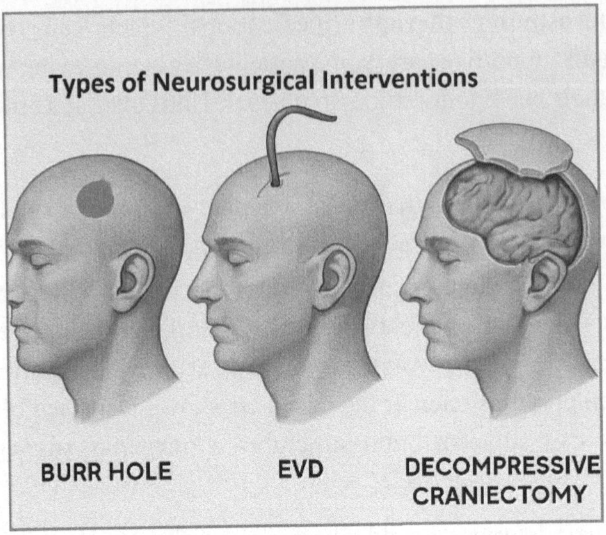

Q6.2.4: Why do some patients deteriorate very quickly after brain haemorrhage?

Sometimes, bleeding occurs in multiple brain areas (e.g., **SAH**) or on one side (e.g., **EDH** or **SDH**). Extra blood raises pressure, compressing vital brain structures. This can lead to **brain herniation** (part of the brain pushing out through the skull base), resulting in loss of functions like breathing, consciousness, and reflexes.

Rarely, patients may become **brain-dead** within a short time despite all protective measures. Recovery from brain injury can be slow, and a sudden intracranial pressure spike may cause deterioration within minutes. To prevent this, patients may be kept on continuous **sedation** while on **ventilator support**. Even excessive coughing or straining during bowel movements can trigger such an event.

In some cases of **diffuse intracranial bleeding** (**SAH**), patients may develop new strokes due to **vasospasm** (sudden narrowing of blood vessels), leading to reduced blood flow to parts of the brain. A patient might initially recover but then show new stroke symptoms despite treatment.

Q6.2.5: Which medical terms are commonly used by doctors when describing the patient's level of consciousness?

- **Alert:** Fully conscious, responds to commands and moves purposefully
- **Disoriented:** Does not recognize place or people
- **Drowsy:** Very sleepy
- **Arousable:** Sleepy but easily awakened
- **Lethargic:** Reduced alertness, slowed thinking due to tiredness
- **Obtunded:** Moderate reduction in alertness
- **Stupor:** Difficult to wake, responds only to pain
- **Delirium:** Awake but confused, with abnormal behaviour
- **Coma:** No voluntary movement, does not respond to stimuli
- **Vegetative State:** Unconscious, but has sleep–wake cycles and may appear awake
- **Brain-dead:** Unconscious, unresponsive, no brainstem functions like breathing, coughing or swallowing
- **Locked-in State:** Completely paralyzed but fully conscious

Doctors frequently refer to **GCS (Glasgow Coma Scale)** to assess consciousness. It is scored between **3 to 15**, based on the patient's response to verbal and painful stimuli (15 = best, 3 = worst).

Patients with **GCS ≤ 8** are considered comatose and may require **intubation** (placement of a breathing tube into the windpipe) and **ventilator support**.

Comatose patients cannot protect their **airway** (breathing tract) and are at high risk of **aspiration pneumonia** (lung infection due to entry of saliva or vomit into the lungs). Hence, intubation is essential to prevent respiratory complications.

Q6.2.6: What is the difference between "coma" and "brain-dead"?

Patient's relatives should understand one important fact: a brain-dead patient is always considered to be in a coma, but not all comatose patients are brain-dead.

Coma is a state of unconsciousness in which a person cannot be awakened by painful stimuli, sound, or light. However, such patients may still have spontaneous breathing efforts along with other preserved brainstem reflexes.

Brainstem reflexes are involuntary motor responses such as coughing, swallowing, sneezing, and breathing.

Some comatose conditions are **reversible** if doctors can correct the underlying cause—for example, metabolic abnormalities (like abnormal levels of glucose, sodium, carbon dioxide, ammonia, or urea) or infections. After appropriate treatment, the patient may come out of a coma.

Some comatose conditions are **irreversible**—for example, extensive brain damage caused by **hypoxic brain injury** (low oxygen reaching the brain), severe bleeding compressing vital brain structures, or a large stroke involving more than half of the brain. These patients may die within a few days or remain in a coma or vegetative state.

The **brainstem**, located in the centre of the brain, plays a vital role in sustaining life. If it is damaged due to stroke or bleeding, patients may not even be able to breathe spontaneously. A person can live with paralysis, but once the brainstem stops functioning, they cannot survive without ventilator support. Even with ventilator assistance, such patients may succumb eventually.

Hence, patients with absent brainstem functions are considered "**brain-dead**." Brain-dead patients may show normal heartbeat and blood pressure, but they cannot breathe on their own and are entirely dependent on ventilatory support.

Q6.2.7: What is the procedure for "brain-death declaration"?

If a patient remains unconscious for more than 24 hours with no movement or response to sound, light, or painful stimuli, and shows no spontaneous breathing efforts, doctors may suspect permanent brainstem damage.

Several tests must be conducted to confirm that the patient is indeed "brain-dead." One key test is the **Apnoea Test** (apnoea means absence of breathing), which helps confirm that the patient cannot breathe spontaneously.

To conduct this test:

- The ventilator is disconnected for a few minutes while oxygen is still provided directly through the breathing tube.
- Doctors perform **ABG (Arterial Blood Gas)** tests before and after the apnoea test to monitor carbon dioxide (CO_2) levels.
- If CO_2 level rises significantly and there are no visible breathing efforts, the first apnoea test is documented as "positive."

A second apnoea test must be performed **six hours** after the first one. If it also yields positive results, based on the two ABG reports, the treating physician—after consulting with two other doctors—can legally declare brain death.

Relatives should understand that the brain-death declaration process may take **few hours** as doctors must rule out all treatable causes of coma first. Additional tests like **CT scan**, **MRI of the brain**, or **EEG (Electroencephalogram)** may be performed alongside the **apnoea test**.

Q6.2.8: What options are available to the patient's family once doctors declare brain death?

After brain death is declared, families may have several questions about next steps. They must choose one of the following options:

a. Consider **end-of-life care** and withdraw ongoing treatment, including removal of ventilator support

b. Consider **organ donation**, only if the family voluntarily consents following brain-death declaration

c. Continue life-support treatment indefinitely (although the patient's heart will eventually stop beating within hours to days despite the life support)

The third option is medically impractical, as there is no chance of recovery once brain death has been confirmed.

Q6.2.9: How do doctors document the "exact time of death" during brain-death declaration?

People often assume a person is considered dead when the heart stops and breathing ceases. However, in medical practice there are **two types of death**:

- **Circulatory Death**: Occurs when the heart stops pumping blood—this is the irreversible end of circulation and breathing.
- **Brain Death**: Occurs when brain activity ceases permanently due to irreversible damage but blood circulation is continuous due to heart pumping activity.

Relatives must understand that normal heart function can persist briefly even after brain death. A patient cannot be declared dead (circulatory death) while the heart is still pumping.

But if brain death is confirmed by two positive apnoea tests spaced six hours apart, the patient is legally dead.

If the family decides to withdraw life support by signing an **end-of-life care** consent form, the ventilator may be removed, leading to cardiac arrest and circulatory death.

The official time of death in brain-death cases is documented as the time of the second apnoea test. Specifically, the time recorded on the second ABG test during that procedure becomes the legal time of death.

Q6.2.10: Why do some patients show sudden arm or leg movements even after brain-death declaration?

Sometimes, brain-dead patients may exhibit sudden hand or leg movements after death declaration. This may cause families to question whether the patient is truly dead or not. This phenomenon can be explained by a rare reflex called the **"Lazarus Sign."** It involves brief arm movements that cross over the chest and occur due to **spinal reflexes**, even in brain-dead patients.

Though disturbing to observe, these movements do not indicate life or potential recovery. Brain-dead patients may also show other spinal reflexes such as:

- **Sudden finger jerks**
- **Muscle stretch reflexes**
- **Plantar responses (upward movement of toes)**

These movements can understandably cause confusion. Families should request medical explanations from doctors before assuming that the patient is still alive. Misunderstandings can lead to unnecessary emotional distress or false accusations against the medical team.

Once brain death is confirmed, recovery is not possible, regardless of such reflex activity.

Q6.2.11: What are the possible outcomes and long-term consequences after severe traumatic brain injury or brain haemorrhage?

Brain haemorrhage or **traumatic brain injury (TBI)** can result in a wide range of short-term and long-term outcomes.

These vary from person to person depending on injury severity, the brain area involved, age, health status, and how quickly treatment is given.

Immediate Outcomes:

- Loss of consciousness (drowsiness, semi-coma, or coma)
- **Cognitive impairments** (e.g., memory loss, problem-solving difficulty)
- **Physical impairments** (e.g., paralysis or weakness)
- **Motor coordination problems** (e.g., ataxia—poor balance and walking)
- **Seizures** (involuntary limb jerking or convulsions)
- **Speech and language problems** (difficulty speaking or understanding)

- **Emotional and behavioural changes** (e.g., mood swings, personality changes)
- **Autonomic dysfunction** (e.g., blood pressure, heart rate, or temperature fluctuations)

Long-Term Consequences:

- Persistent cognitive deficits
- Motor and sensory impairments
- Ongoing speech and language issues
- Psychological and behavioural disorders
- Chronic pain (e.g., in the head, neck, or back)
- Recurrent seizures or epilepsy
- **Hydrocephalus** (accumulation of cerebrospinal fluid in the brain)
- Progressive neurodegeneration and dementia
- Lasting disability and reduced quality of life

Relatives should understand that while some patients recover completely, others may become permanently bedbound and live with disabilities. Recovery may range from full independence to ongoing challenges that significantly impact quality of life.

Diagnosis: 6.3 CVST (Cerebral Venous Sinus Thrombosis)

Cerebral venous sinus thrombosis (CVST) is a condition in which a blood clot forms in the venous sinuses of the brain, blocking blood flow and leading to increased intracranial (inside the skull) pressure.

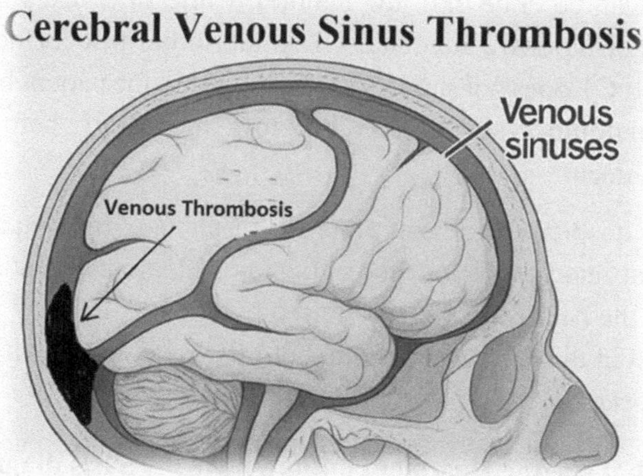

The venous sinuses are important structures responsible for draining deoxygenated blood from the brain back to the heart.

Most common causes of CVST:

- Prothrombotic conditions (conditions that increase the tendency of blood to clot)
- Hormonal imbalance (pregnancy, oral contraceptive pills, hormone therapy)
- Infections of the ear, sinuses, or brain
- Head injury
- Dehydration
- Cancer

The symptoms of CVST vary depending on the location of the clot and severity of the blockage. Common symptoms include headache, seizures, visual disturbances, altered consciousness, confusion, or memory loss.

Q6.3.1: Why do doctors advise an MRI of the brain even if a CT scan has already been done?

CT scan of the brain is a good tool for detecting bleeding but is less effective at identifying venous sinus thrombosis. MRI provides detailed information about venous sinuses. If blood is not flowing freely through any sinus, MRI can detect it clearly.

A CT scan can be done in a few minutes, while MRI takes longer. If a patient cannot lie down for long, CT is the initial test for neurological symptoms. If CT does not show major findings but the patient has a severe headache and other signs, MRI becomes mandatory before starting specific treatment.

Since many hospitals do not have an MRI machine in-house, patients may need to visit another diagnostic centre for MRI scan. Relatives should understand the necessity of tests advised by doctors. CT may be the first imaging test in the emergency room, but MRI might be required later for final diagnosis.

Q6.3.2: What are the treatment options once CVST is diagnosed?

Anticoagulation therapy: To prevent clot growth and allow natural breakdown. Patients receive injections (e.g., Heparin) after MRI confirmation. These are later replaced with oral anticoagulant tablets for long-term use (3–6 months).

Thrombolysis (clot-busting therapy): In severe cases with significant swelling or neurological decline, thrombolytic agents (e.g., tissue plasminogen activator injection) may be used to dissolve the clot.

Neurosurgery: Rarely, surgery may be needed to remove the clot or relieve brain pressure if thrombolysis is not effective or safe.

Treating underlying conditions (e.g., infections or clotting disorders) and symptomatic management (e.g., anti-seizure injections, therapies to reduce brain pressure) is crucial.

Q6.3.3: What are the possible outcomes after CVST?

Prognosis varies based on clot extent, speed of diagnosis, and treatment effectiveness:

- **Good prognosis**: With early diagnosis and anticoagulation, many patients recover fully or with minimal residual effects.
- **Poor prognosis**: If severe brain damage occurs or complications like stroke or brain herniation develop, permanent disability or death may result.

Q6.3.4: How can someone prevent CVST?

At-risk individuals (e.g., cancer patients, pregnant women, patients with clotting disorders, women on oral contraceptives or hormonal therapy) should:

- Maintain adequate hydration to prevent blood thickening and clot formation
- Treat any underlying conditions or infections promptly
- Avoid smoking, as cessation helps reduce risk

Diagnosis: 6.4 Meningitis

Meningitis is an infection of the protective outer membranes (meninges) surrounding the brain and spinal cord.

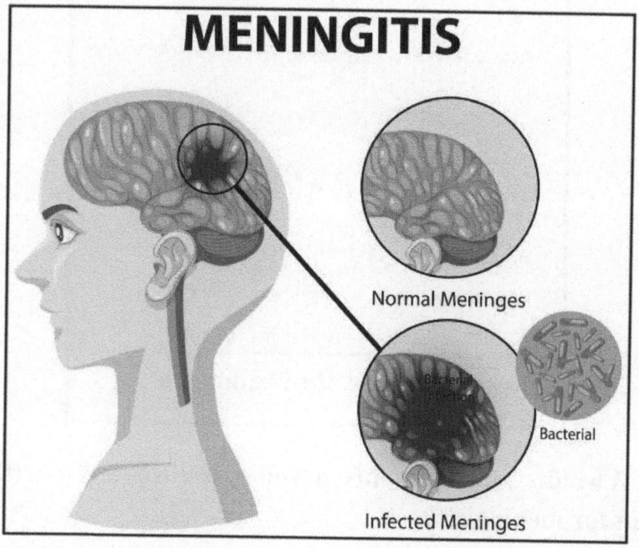

It can be caused by bacteria, viruses, fungi, or other organisms. Symptoms include fever, severe headache, stiff neck, nausea, vomiting, light sensitivity, confusion, or seizures.

Infants, young children, and older adults are particularly vulnerable.

Q6.4.1: What investigations are advised when meningitis is suspected?

Beyond clinical signs (e.g., fever, headache, stiff neck), additional tests include:

- **Lumbar puncture (spinal tap)**: CSF (cerebrospinal fluid) is collected to check for infection and determine type (bacterial, viral, fungal, etc.)
- **Blood tests**: To detect infection
- **Imaging**: CT or MRI to rule out other conditions causing similar symptoms
- **Multiplex PCR test**: Advanced test that detects multiple organisms in body fluids using **Polymerase Chain Reaction (PCR)** technology

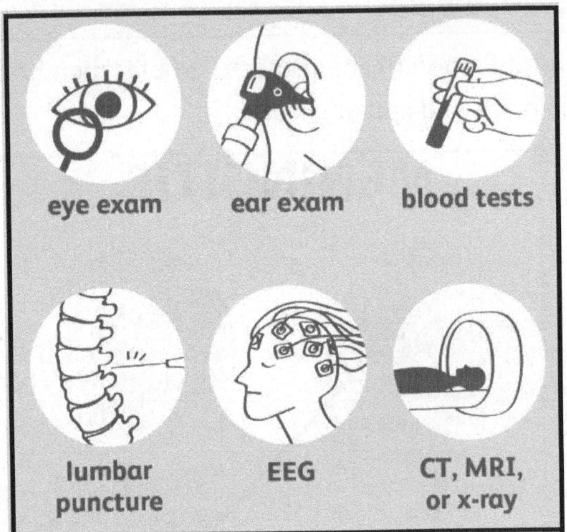

Investigations for Meningitis

Q6.4.2: Why do some patients develop seizures even with proper treatment for meningitis?

Seizure refers to involuntary body movements, sometimes called "fits."

Seizures occur when normal brain function is disrupted due to infection, swelling, or increased pressure. Seizures related to meningitis don’t necessarily mean the patient has or will develop **epilepsy** (a condition causing recurrent seizures).

They may also result from **metabolic disturbances** like low glucose or sodium. Even with proper treatment, changes can occur in the brain during the first 4–5 days.

Relatives should know that seizures may happen during ICU care despite effective treatment. Some patients may experience repeated seizures requiring multiple medications. If the patient doesn't regain full consciousness between episodes, it is called **status epilepticus**.

In some cases, the patient may not show jerky movements but may still have **silent seizures**, staying unconscious or semi-conscious. To detect this, **EEG (Electroencephalogram)**—a test that records brain activity using scalp electrodes—is used. Doctors may refer to this condition as **NCSE (Non-Convulsive Status Epilepticus)**. Continuous EEG monitoring may be needed to adjust treatment.

Prolonged seizures can cause brain injury and coma.

Q6.4.3: What are possible outcomes for patients with meningitis?

Outcomes depend on factors like age, health status, immunity, and disease severity:

- **Bacterial meningitis**: If treated early with appropriate antibiotics, recovery can begin within 4–5 days, provided no severe complications like seizures or brain pressure occur
- **Viral meningitis**: Mostly requires supportive care; many viral infections resolve on their own. Antiviral injections may sometimes be used.
- While many patients recover after extended ICU care, some may develop permanent brain damage due to pressure or low oxygen delivery, leading to coma or death

Q6.4.4: What is encephalitis? Can meningitis and encephalitis occur together?

Encephalitis is brain inflammation usually caused by a viral infection. There are two main types:

- **Infectious encephalitis**: Caused by viruses, including those spread by mosquitoes or ticks
- **Autoimmune encephalitis**: Caused by the immune system mistakenly attacking brain tissue

Meningoencephalitis occurs when the brain and meninges are inflamed simultaneously. It can result from bacteria, viruses, fungi, or parasites. This condition is life-threatening and may lead to death even with treatment, particularly if brain damage is severe.

Diagnosis: 6.5 Pneumonia

Pneumonia is an infection of the lungs that causes symptoms like cough and breathing difficulty. The small air sacs of the lungs (**alveoli**) become filled with fluid and other secretions, causing a drop of oxygen levels in the blood.

Not all patients with pneumonia require hospitalization, but doctors may recommend ICU admission if oxygen saturation is low or if the patient's vitals (blood pressure, heart rate, etc.) are unstable.

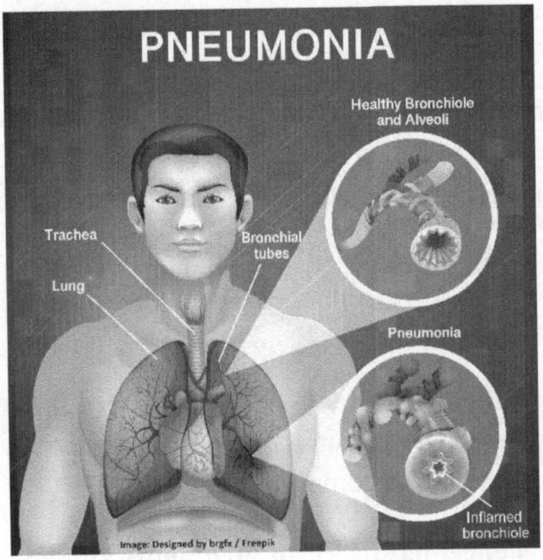

Doctors may use specific terminology for different types of pneumonia:

- **Community-Acquired Pneumonia** (if the patient develops pneumonia at home)
- **Hospital-Acquired Pneumonia** (if pneumonia develops after 2 days of hospital admission)
- **Aspiration Pneumonia** (due to inhalation of food, liquid, or vomit into the lungs because of altered consciousness or difficulty swallowing)

- **Ventilator-Associated Pneumonia** (if pneumonia occurs in patients on mechanical ventilation for more than 48 hours)

Q6.5.1: What investigations may be required if a patient is suspected to have pneumonia?

- **Chest X-ray** (may be repeated to monitor disease progress)
- **HRCT Chest** (High-Resolution Computed Tomography)
- **CBP (Complete Blood Picture)**: assesses white blood cell count, which may be elevated during severe infection
- **RFT (Renal Function Test)**: includes creatinine, urea, and electrolytes
- **ABG (Arterial Blood Gas)**: assesses oxygen and carbon dioxide levels, and acid-base status
- **Blood and Sputum Culture–Sensitivity**: identifies the causative organism

These are minimum tests needed for ICU-admitted pneumonia patients.

If the condition worsens, leading to intubation and mechanical ventilation, further tests may be needed:

- **Bronchoscopy**: removes mucus plugs from bronchi and helps collect secretions for lab analysis
- **Multiplex PCR Test**: detects multiple microorganisms in body fluids or blood using **Polymerase Chain Reaction (PCR)** technology

Q6.5.2: How can relatives know whether pneumonia is resolving?

- The best method is by **chest X-ray**. Sometimes, the patient may clinically improve within 4–5 days, but the X-ray might still show abnormal findings.
- Doctors usually explain progress based on the patient's **oxygen requirement** and **breathing parameters**.

- For example: if the patient required 10 litres of oxygen per minute upon admission and later needs only 2 litres per minute, this suggests improvement.
- For patients who are on ventilator support, relatives can observe the requirement of oxygen percentage from ventilator to have some idea about lung recovery.

Two Parameters on the ventilator screen can give information about patient's ventilator support:

- **FiO_2 (Fraction of Inspired Oxygen)**
- **PEEP (Positive End-Expiratory Pressure)**

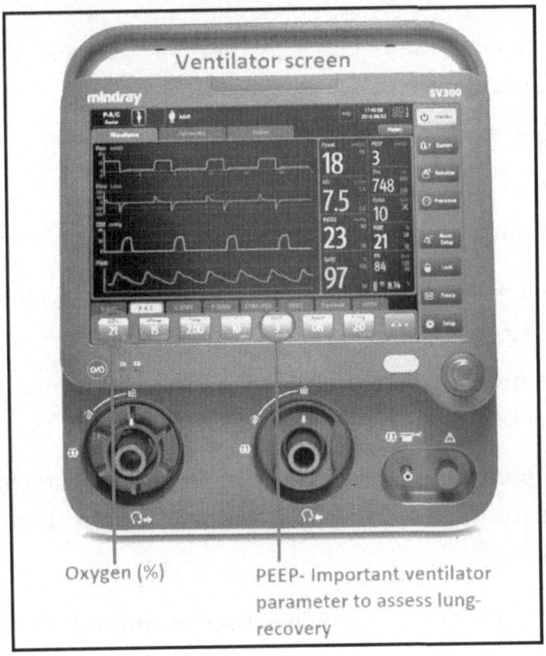

Normal air contains 21% oxygen. In pneumonia, initially patients may be ventilated with 100% oxygen (Fio2=100% and gradually oxygen concentration may be reduced to 30–40% as the patient improves.

- **PEEP** is the residual pressure in the lungs after exhalation, used to keep alveoli open.

If the patient initially needed high PEEP (10–14) and later maintains good oxygen levels with reduced PEEP (5–8), this also indicates recovery.

Q6.5.3: What are the treatment options if oxygen levels do not improve, even with ventilator support?

In severe pneumonia, **oxygen therapy** is critical:

- Initially, oxygen may be given via nasal cannula.
- If ineffective, doctors may escalate to:
    - Face mask
    - Non-rebreathing mask (with attached reservoir bag)
    - HFNC (High-Flow Nasal Cannula)
    - NIV (Non-Invasive Ventilation mask)

If oxygen saturation remains persistently low, the patient may get **intubated** and connected to a **ventilator**. Most patients improve with ventilator support, but in some cases, oxygen levels remain low even at maximum ventilatory settings.

In such cases, options are limited:

➢ **Prone Ventilation**: Patient is kept in lying face-down position with ongoing invasive mechanical ventilator support to improve oxygen level.

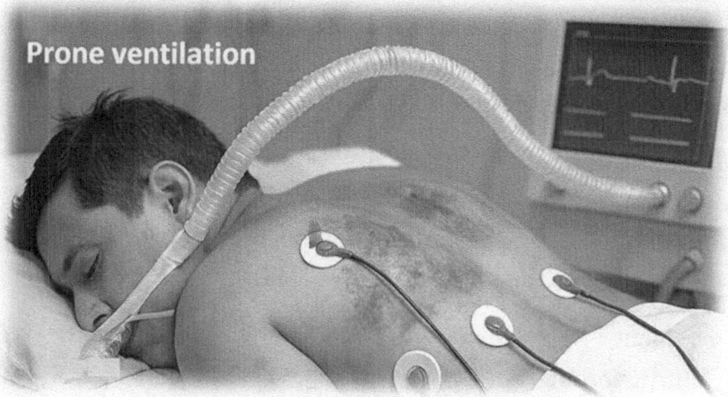

➢ **ECMO (Extracorporeal Membrane Oxygenation)**: Patient's blood is oxygenated outside the body using a pump and membrane (with help of ECMO machine) till the lungs recover from pneumonia.

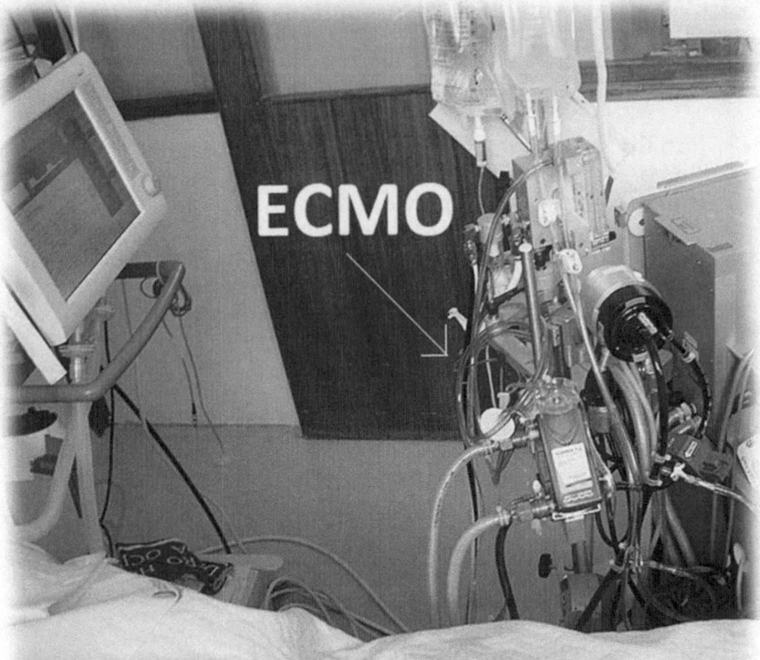

Image By Cmenesesoliveira - Own work, Public Domain, https://commons.wikimedia.org/w/index.php?curid=9044324

Q6.5.4: When, why, and for how long is prone ventilation needed in severe pneumonia?

If oxygen saturation remains below 92% despite 100% oxygen from ventilator, **prone ventilation** may help.

Alveoli in the lungs are not evenly ventilated. In a supine (face-up) position, front lung regions are better ventilated, while back areas may remain collapsed. Prone position helps open alveoli in the back of the lungs, improving oxygenation.

- Patient is kept unconscious and immobile with **sedative drugs** during prone ventilation.
- If oxygen levels improve, sessions may last **16–24 hours**.
- After each session, the patient is returned to supine position for 4–6 hours.

- If improvement continues, further prone sessions (total 3–5) may be needed.
- Once oxygen saturation stays above 92% in supine position, prone ventilation can be stopped.

Key Points to remember for Patient's Relatives During Prone Ventilation:

- There will be always a risk of **sudden cardiac arrest** if oxygen levels do not improve even after keeping patient in prone position
- Prone ventilation is feasible **only if blood pressure and heart rhythm are stable**
- **Swelling of the eyes, lips, and tongue** may occur due to prolonged face-down positioning but this swelling will reduce with recovery
- **Skin injuries** may occur due to pressure; eye injuries are also possible despite precautions
- Doctors prioritize **oxygenation and survival** over temporary physical appearance
- **Some patients may still deteriorate or die**, despite appropriate ventilation and prone therapy
- Recovery depends on **multiple factors**, and pneumonia may be fatal in severe cases—even with full ICU support

Q6.5.5: When does a patient with severe pneumonia need ECMO (Extracorporeal Membrane Oxygenation), and what basic information should the patient's relatives know?

ECMO is considered the last resort for patients with severe pneumonia when all other interventions fail to improve oxygenation. If the patient's oxygen saturation does not increase even after initiating ventilator support and prone ventilation, doctors may recommend ECMO to improve oxygenation. ECMO is advised for patients with extensive pneumonia (visible on HRCT chest scan) and severe hypoxia (low oxygen in the body), which can be assessed by ABG (Arterial Blood Gas) analysis.

ECMO is a **high-cost therapy**, and not all hospitals have the necessary facilities and teams to provide it. Patients may need to be shifted to a hospital where ECMO is available, or an ECMO team may be called to initiate support at the bedside. In such cases, ECMO can be continued during ambulance transport to the higher centre.

ECMO can support both the **lungs and the heart**, and the type of ECMO support is determined based on patient condition:

VV-ECMO (Veno-Venous): used when only the lungs are affected

VA-ECMO (Veno-Arterial): used when both the lungs and heart are severely compromised or if heart function is very weak with significant low blood pressure.

Most patients with severe pneumonia benefit from VV-ECMO; however, those with critically low blood pressure may require VA-ECMO.

During the initial days of ECMO, patients may require deep sedation. Later, if they breathe comfortably with ventilator and ECMO support, sedation may be reduced. **Weaning from ECMO** (reducing ECMO support very slowly) is a gradual process and may take days to weeks depending on lung recovery.

ECMO treatment is expensive, and since the **duration of therapy is unpredictable**, not all families can afford it. In some cases, patient's relatives have to take difficult decisions regarding the **withdrawal of ECMO support** due to financial constraints if patient's clinical condition doesn't show any major improvement.

If oxygen levels remain poor despite ECMO, **prone ventilation along with ECMO** may be recommended as a last attempt to improve oxygenation.

ECMO can lead to **complications** such as bleeding or blood clot formation, which can delay recovery. In such cases, doctors may need to replace the oxygenator membrane if membrane starts showing any blood clots and this may add to treatment costs.

If lung recovery is slow and the patient remains dependent on ECMO, families must remain patient and hopeful. Many patients with severe pneumonia have recovered even after **6–8 weeks** of ECMO support.

Patients with pneumonia and **hypoxemia** (low blood oxygen) are prone to develop sudden cardiac arrest. Even on ECMO, deterioration may occur quickly if cardiac arrest happens. Hence, families should understand that **death may still occur** despite ECMO support if patient is extremely critical.

Q6.5.6: What is the average duration for recovery from severe pneumonia?

Patients with severe pneumonia may begin to recover within **6 to 7 days** if their lungs respond quickly to treatment.

If ventilator support is required, full recovery may take **2 to 3 weeks**, assuming no major complications.

If a **tracheostomy** is needed for prolonged ventilation, ICU stay may extend beyond **3 to 4 weeks**.

Some patients develop **critical illness polyneuropathy (CIP)**—extreme muscle weakness and nerve damage due to prolonged ICU care. Such patients may need further rehabilitation for few weeks.

Families should understand that **no exact timeline exists** for recovery from severe illness. Repeatedly asking doctors for a fixed duration for recovery may not be helpful.

Q6.5.7: What kind of clinical course can be expected in a patient with severe pneumonia?

There are 3 **possible outcomes** in severe pneumonia:

a) Early Recovery

- If lungs improve quickly with antibiotics, patient's oxygen requirement may get reduced day by day.
- The patient **may not need ventilator support**, recover within **5–6 days**, and be discharged home without oxygen.

b) Late Recovery

- If oxygen requirement increases in the first few days, ventilator support may be necessary.

- If ventilation continues beyond **5–6 days, tracheostomy** (tube placed via a small neck incision) may be advised.
- These patients usually recover slowly over weeks and may be discharged to a **rehabilitation centre**, often with minimal oxygen support.
- Those with **multi-organ involvement** may need extended ICU stay before full recovery.

c) Mortality (Death Despite Treatment)

- A small number of patients may have **critically low oxygen levels** even with 100% oxygen support from the ventilator.
- These patients are at risk of **sudden cardiac arrest** during treatment.
- If prone ventilation or ECMO is required, families should be prepared for the possibility of unexpected deterioration, even with appropriate treatment.

Diagnosis: 6.6 COPD (Chronic Obstructive Pulmonary Disease)

Chronic Obstructive Pulmonary Disease (COPD) is a progressive lung condition that makes breathing difficult due to obstruction in the airflow through the lungs and airways.

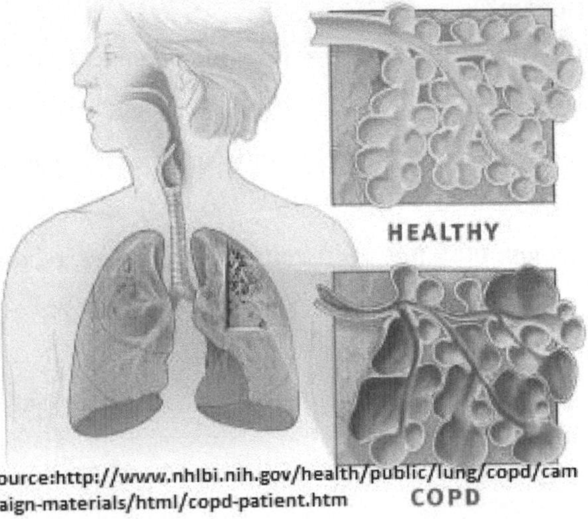

Source:http://www.nhlbi.nih.gov/health/public/lung/copd/campaign-materials/html/copd-patient.htm

It commonly affects smokers and individuals exposed to environmental pollutants through their occupation. Permanent changes in the lungs gradually reduce lung function, and patients may require frequent ICU admissions.

Q6.6.1: What is 'Acute Exacerbation of COPD' (AECOPD)?

AECOPD refers to an episode of sudden worsening of COPD symptoms caused by infection, exposure to pollutants, or seasonal changes.

Many patients require ICU admission during an AECOPD episode due to respiratory failure.

Q6.6.2: When does a COPD patient need ICU admission?

ICU admission may be necessary if any of the following abnormal findings are present:

- Excessively high respiratory rate (more than 30 breaths per minute) despite nebulisation and other treatments
- **Respiratory failure**:
    - **Type 1**: Low oxygen in blood
    - **Type 2**: High carbon dioxide in blood
- **Acidosis**: A blood pH < 7.35 due to carbon dioxide retention
- **Altered mental status** from low oxygen (**hypoxia**) or high carbon dioxide (**hypercapnia**)—patients may become irritable or excessively drowsy
- **Unstable vitals**, including low blood pressure and irregular heart rhythms
- **Inability to protect the airway**—unconscious patients unable to swallow may aspirate, increasing pneumonia risk if stomach content or oral secretions enter the lungs
- **Persistent NIV (Non-Invasive Ventilation) support**

- **Intubation** and **initiation of invasive ventilator support** in the emergency room

Q6.6.3: How do doctors treat critically ill COPD patients in the ICU?

Treatment of COPD patients in ICU focuses on four major goals:

- **Improve oxygen levels**: COPD patients don't need high oxygen saturation. Even 1–2 litres of oxygen may help maintain SpO_2 (oxygen saturation) between 89% and 92%.

- **Reduce respiratory distress**: Using nebulisations and medications like **bronchodilators** and **systemic steroids** to dilate airways

- **Ensure adequate ventilation**: By providing NIV (non-invasive ventilation) support to help maintain oxygen and carbon dioxide within normal ranges

- **Treat the underlying cause** of exacerbation—typically with **antibiotics** or **antiviral agents**

Q6.6.4: What complications may occur in COPD patients in the ICU?

Loss of consciousness: Often caused by excessive carbon dioxide retention. Many COPD patients need intubation and mechanical ventilation to maintain adequate gas exchange.

Pneumothorax: Air leakage into the pleural cavity due to high-pressure ventilator support, compressing the lungs. An **ICD (Intercostal Drain)** may be required to remove trapped air.

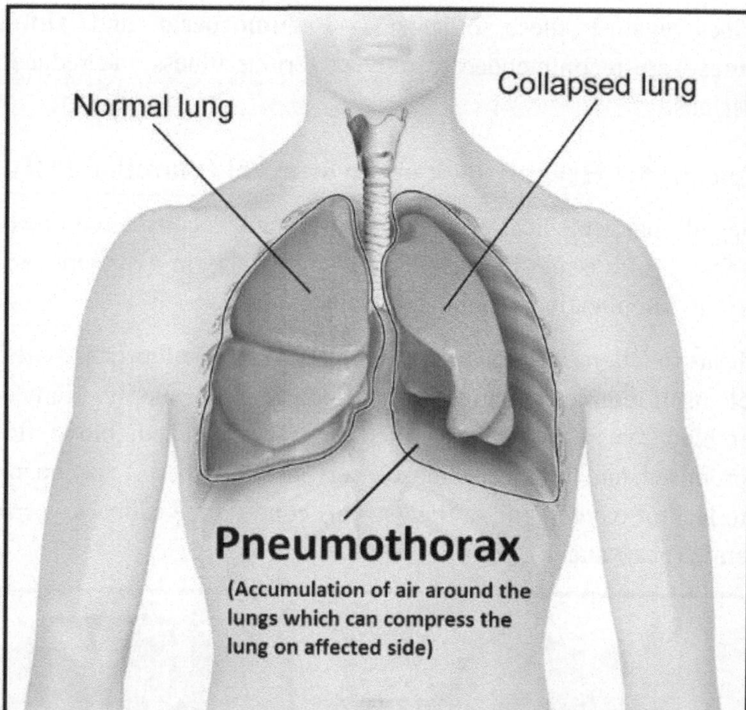

Blausen.com staff (2014). "Medical gallery of Blausen Medical 2014". WikiJournal of Medicine

Lung collapse: Accumulated secretions may block distal airways, preventing air from reaching certain lung areas. This may require **bronchoscopy and lavage** (procedure to clean major airways and bronchus) to clear mucus plugs.

Hypotension: Sudden drop in blood pressure can occur after initiating invasive ventilation.

Subcutaneous emphysema: Air collection under the skin due to high-pressure ventilator support. This may cause noticeable swelling on the face, neck, and chest.

Q6.6.5: Why do doctors advise specific vaccines for COPD patients?

Patients with COPD are prone to frequent infections, especially **pneumonia** and **lower respiratory tract infections**.

Influenza and **pneumococcus** are common pathogens in elderly COPD patients.

Vaccines against these organisms—**Pneumococcal** and **Influenza vaccines**—are recommended to prevent serious illness and reduce ICU admissions.

Diagnosis: 6.7 Heart Attack or Myocardial Infarction (MI)

Among all major medical problems, heart attack is considered one of the most fatal health issues because even a slight delay in treatment can lead to serious complications, including death.

The heart functions as a pump that supplies blood to all organs. The heart muscle itself requires continuous and adequate blood supply. If any of the major blood vessels supplying the heart gets blocked, blood flow is compromised, and the cardiac muscle served by that vessel may be injured due to lack of oxygen and nutrients. This condition is called **myocardial ischemia** (heart attack).

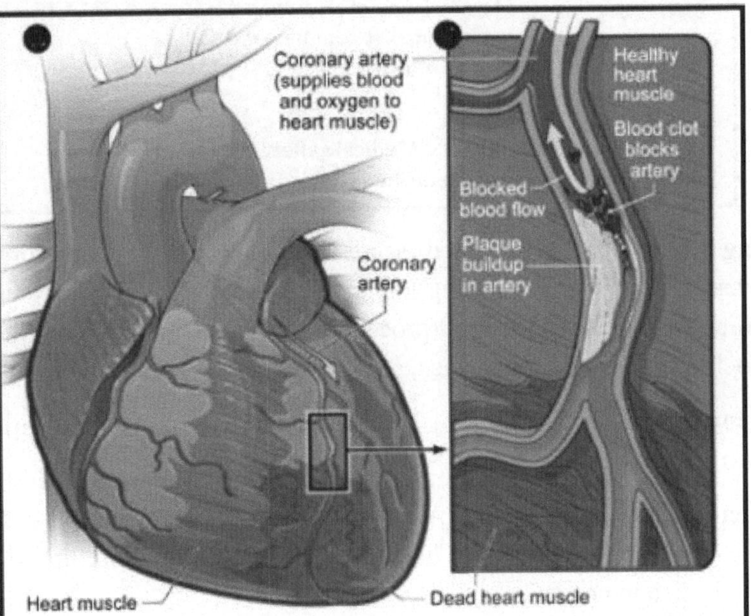

http://www.nhlbi.nih.gov/health/health-topics/topics/heartattack/

When blood supply to a part of the heart is suddenly interrupted, patients may feel **chest pain or discomfort**, which may radiate to the left arm or jaw. Some patients may not experience sharp pain but may describe a **persistent burning sensation** in the middle of the chest.

Q6.7.1: How do doctors diagnose a heart attack?

When a patient presents with chest pain, the first test in the emergency room is an **ECG (Electrocardiogram)**. If ECG findings are abnormal, doctors may check **cardiac markers** (blood test which helps to detect heart attack)—specifically **Troponin-I or Troponin-T levels**. If heart muscle damage occurs due to poor blood supply, cardiac markers are released into the bloodstream within minutes to hours. Elevated troponin confirms the diagnosis. Sometimes, an initial troponin test may be negative if the test is done too early, and the doctor will repeat the same test after a few hours.

To further evaluate the heart, a **2D-ECHO (echocardiography)** may be performed to check the heart's pumping function and muscle movement. Abnormal findings may prompt an invasive procedure called **Coronary Angiogram (CAG)** to assess blood vessel patency.

Tests commonly advised when heart attack is suspected:

- ECG (Electrocardiogram)
- Troponin levels
- 2D-ECHO
- Coronary Angiogram (CAG)

Q6.7.2: What other conditions can cause chest pain besides heart attack?

Chest pain can result from multiple causes. If ECG, 2D-ECHO, and cardiac markers are normal, coronary angiography may not be required immediately. There are many other conditions which can cause chest pain.

- Severe acidity (gastritis)
- Stomach ulcers
- Gastroesophageal reflux (acid movement from stomach to oesophagus/food pipe)
- Gall bladder infection
- Pancreatic infection

- Hernia (gap in chest wall causing abdominal contents to migrate upward)
- Pregnancy
- Muscle strain

Q6.7.3: What are the treatment options for heart attack?

Once a heart attack is suspected, the patient may receive:

- **Two antiplatelet drugs** (blood thinners to prevent clot formation)
- A **statin drug** (to lower cholesterol and lipoproteins)
- Possibly an **anticoagulant injection** (e.g., Heparin) until definitive treatment is done
- **Vasodilator drug** (tablet or injection which helps to increase blood flow to heart muscle by dilating the blood vessels)

The **main treatment goal** is **revascularization**—means restoring blood flow to the heart muscle. This can be achieved through one of these 3 interventions:

(1) Thrombolysis (clot-busting injection):

Used when the hospital lacks a Cath-lab facility. It's effective if the clot is recent. This injection is given in ER (emergency room) and it is very costly injection which can cause bleeding complications too. The patient must eventually be shifted to a Cath-lab-equipped hospital for a coronary angiogram.

(2) Stenting or Balloon Dilatation:

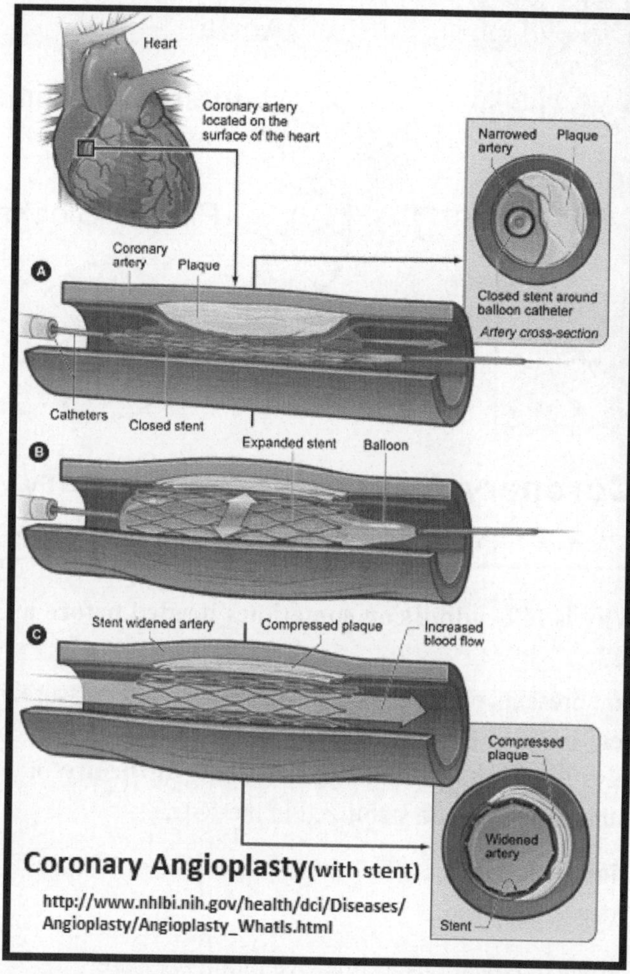

It is known as **PCI (Percutaneous Coronary Intervention)**. A stent is placed in a narrowed vessel to restore blood flow. In multivessel disease, balloon dilatation may be done to open blocked arteries along with stent placement.

This life-saving procedure is done by interventional cardiologist.

(3) Bypass Surgery (CABG - Coronary Artery Bypass Graft): Advised when stenting is not possible due to extensive blockages. CABG operation is performed by a cardiothoracic surgeon.

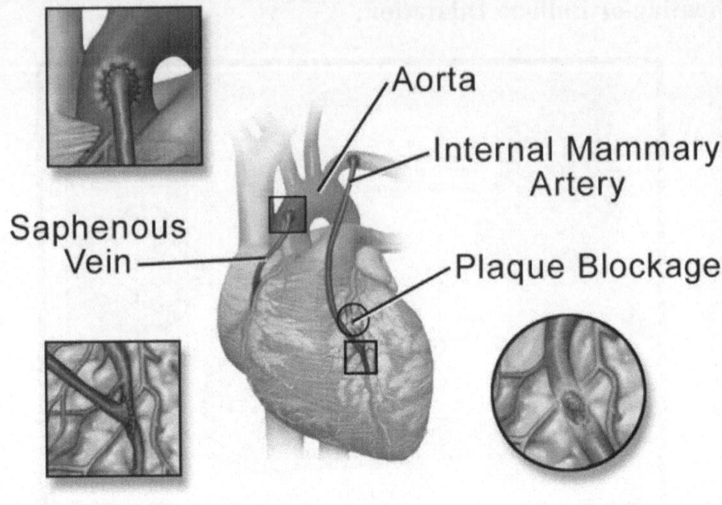

Coronary Artery Bypass Surgery

https://commons.wikimedia.org/wiki/File:Blausen_0151_CABG_02.png

Q6.7.4: Why is ICU admission sometimes needed before a Cath-Lab procedure?

If the patient presents with stable vitals (normal blood pressure, heart rate, and oxygen levels), CAG (Coronary Angiogram) can be performed immediately. But if the patient has **breathing difficulty** or **low blood pressure**, they must first be stabilized in the ICU.

Stabilization includes:

- Oxygen support
- Cardiac medications to improve blood pressure
- NIV (non-invasive ventilation) support if **pulmonary edema** is present (pulmonary edema means excessive fluid accumulation in the lungs due to poor pumping capacity of heart)

Patients must lie flat and remain still on the Cath-lab table for 30 minutes to 2 hours. If they are breathing rapidly or doing constant movements because of chest pain or discomfort, the procedure becomes unsafe. Cardiologists require stable vitals to conduct safe coronary intervention.

In some cases, when chest pain is severe, the cardiologist may proceed with CAG (Coronary Angiogram) despite unstable vitals if delay could worsen the condition.

Q6.7.5: What complications can occur after a heart attack despite treatment?

Even after timely and appropriate intervention, complications may arise, including:

- Bleeding
- Arrhythmias (irregular heart rhythms)
- Vasovagal episodes (sudden drop in blood pressure and heart rate)
- Heart failure (due to reduced pumping ability)
- Pericarditis or Dressler Syndrome (inflammation of the heart's outer lining)
- Reinfarction (second heart attack)
- Stent thrombosis (new blood clot formation in the stented area despite blood thinners)
- Heart muscle rupture, which can lead to cardiac arrest and sudden death

Q6.7.6: What Is an IABP (Intra-Aortic Balloon Pump) and Why Is It Used?

An **IABP- Intra-Aortic Balloon Pump** is a mechanical device that increases blood flow to the heart muscle and reduces the workload on the heart. It involves placing a **catheter with a balloon** via the groin into a major artery. The balloon inflates and deflates with each heartbeat, improving coronary perfusion and cardiac output.

IABP is used temporarily (for hours to days) in patients with:

- **Cardiogenic shock** (persistent low blood pressure after heart attack)
- **High-risk cardiac conditions** requiring non-cardiac surgery or PCI (percutaneous coronary intervention means stenting or balloon angioplasty)

- **Low cardiac output after bypass surgery**

When medications (vasopressors and inotropes) are insufficient to maintain blood pressure and pumping function of heart, IABP helps stabilize vitals until recovery.

Q6.7.7: What are the possible outcomes if a patient requires CPR (Cardiopulmonary Resuscitation) before coronary angioplasty?

Most patients with heart attack arrive at the hospital with chest pain, but a few may become unconscious on the way to hospital or in the emergency department due to cardiac arrest caused by arrhythmias (extremely high or low heart rate).

CPR must be started immediately if the patient is unresponsive with absent pulse and should be continued until pulse or consciousness is restored. Many patients may need **DC shock** (direct current shock) via defibrillator during CPR.

If cardiac arrest occurs, it becomes difficult to predict recovery. Some patients may not respond even after **prolonged CPR** (more than 20–30 minutes), and death must be declared after recording flat-line ECG.

If CPR lasts only for a short duration (2–5 minutes), the patient may regain consciousness quickly and should be shifted to the **Cath-lab** for **CAG (Coronary Angiogram)**. If significant blockages are found, **angioplasty** (stenting or balloon dilatation) is performed to restore blood flow.

If cardiac activity returns after **prolonged CPR** and the patient remains unconscious, doctors consider the possibility of **irreversible brain damage** due to poor oxygen supply during CPR. Such patients are placed on **ventilator support** and **observation** for 24 hours to assess brain function.

Cardiologists usually do **not recommend Cath-lab procedures (stenting or balloon angioplasty)** for unconscious patients who required prolonged CPR, as performing angioplasty may be meaningless if brain recovery is unlikely.

Prognosis depends on several factors:

- **Duration of CPR**: Short CPR (2–5 minutes) with full consciousness has better outcomes than prolonged CPR (>10–15 minutes)
- **Location of arrest**: Outcomes are poorer if cardiac arrest occurs at home or in transit to the hospital.
- **Number of episodes**: Multiple episodes of arrest before or during angioplasty lead to poor outcomes.

Q6.7.8: When do doctors recommend ECMO (Extracorporeal Membrane Oxygenation) for cardiac patients?

ECMO is a life-support machine (heart-lung machine) that temporarily takes over the function of the heart and lungs. It is very costly life-support which can cause bleeding complications too. Patient must fulfil eligibility criteria to receive ECMO because it is not suitable treatment option for every patient.

In cardiac patients, if the heart fails to pump adequately due to heart attack or other causes, it may lead to **cardiogenic shock** (persistently low blood pressure secondary to heart dysfunction). **VA-ECMO (Veno-Arterial ECMO)** is used for cardiac support in the following conditions:

- Sudden worsening of **chronic heart failure**
- **Heart attack** with low BP even after stenting
- **Pulmonary embolism** (major lung vessel blocked by a clot, reducing blood flow to the heart)
- Support after **heart transplant**
- **Drug overdose** that impairs heart function
- **Septic cardiomyopathy** (infection-related cardiac failure)
- **Refractory ventricular tachycardia** (ineffective pumping due to extremely fast heart rate)
- **Cardiac arrest**: In rare cases, ECMO can be initiated during CPR (**eCPR-** Extracorporeal Cardiopulmonary Resuscitation) if the hospital has the required setup and team

Q6.7.9: When is PCI (Percutaneous Coronary Intervention) or stenting advised?

Coronary stenting is essential in most heart attack cases but is also recommended in certain non-emergency conditions.

Patients may need PCI/stent in the following scenarios:

- **Heart attack** with significant vessel blockage causing blood flow obstruction to heart muscles
- **Exertional chest pain or breathlessness** (e.g., while running or climbing stairs), with coronary artery narrowing
- **Silent disease**: Asymptomatic patients with abnormal ECG or 2D ECHO findings may need CAG (coronary angiogram) and stenting
- **Positive treadmill test (TMT)**, followed by CAG indicating significant vessel narrowing
- **Preoperative cardiac evaluation**: Patients scheduled for major surgery may undergo **dobutamine stress echocardiography** (echo is done after giving a drug which can increase heart rates) if unable to do treadmill testing. If heart function declines with stress, further assessment with CAG may be needed, and PCI may be advised before elective surgery.

Q6.7.10: Why might a cardiologist recommend CABG surgery instead of stenting?

CABG (Coronary Artery Bypass Graft) may be advised when stenting isn't feasible due to the nature or extent of coronary disease. Cardiologists may refer patients to cardiothoracic surgeons for CABG surgery based on CAG (coronary angiogram) findings.

CABG may be recommended for:

- **Triple vessel disease** (blockage in all three major coronary arteries)
- **Left main coronary artery blockage**
- **Significant two-vessel disease** with **proximal LAD** (left anterior descending artery) involvement

Sometimes stenting may not be possible due to **anatomical abnormalities** or **technical challenges**. In cases of **failed PTCA** (Percutaneous Transluminal Coronary Angioplasty- invasive procedure in which stent is placed in the coronary vessels to establish adequate blood flow), CABG can be considered for revascularization.

Q6.7.11: How long does a patient need to stay in hospital after a heart attack?

If the patient undergoes **coronary stenting**, cardiac monitoring is needed for **36–48 hours**. If there are no major complications after the procedure, patients can be discharged within **2 days**. Post-discharge, regular **antiplatelet medication** must be taken by patients to prevent stent blockage.

If stenting is not possible and the patient undergoes **CABG** surgery, patient has to stay in hospital for **4–5 days** if there aren't any postoperative complications.

Since cardiac patients are prone to have sudden changes in vitals, **the exact duration of hospitalization** may vary, especially if complications arise after stenting or surgery.

Diagnosis: 6.8 Heart Failure

Heart failure is a chronic (long-standing) condition in which the heart does not pump adequately. If the pumping function is affected suddenly, it is referred to as **acute heart failure**, which may occur due to a heart attack **(myocardial infarction)** or extremely high blood pressure **(hypertensive heart failure).**

There are two main types of heart failure:

- **Systolic heart failure**: Type of heart failure in which the heart cannot pump blood effectively.
- **Diastolic heart failure**: In this type of heart failure, the heart does not relax adequately leading to inadequate filling of its chambers.

Common signs of heart failure include shortness of breath, swollen legs, facial swelling, and fatigue. Some patients experience significant breathing difficulty at night when lying flat leading to **disturbed sleep** and **night-time breathlessness.**

The primary goal of treatment is to reduce the workload on the heart by controlling **fluid volume in the body**. Patients often need daily medications such as:

- **Diuretics** (drugs to produce more urine and reduce fluid overload)
- **Heart rate–controlling drugs**

There is no permanent cure for heart failure except **heart transplantation,** which may not be suitable for all patients. When extra stress is placed on the heart, **pulmonary edema** (fluid accumulation in the lungs) may occur due to poor pumping or relaxation. This leads to **low oxygen levels** and requires **ICU admission**, **oxygen therapy**, **diuretic injections** (medicine which increases urine production), and possibly **breathing support**.

Q6.8.1: What are the signs of worsening heart failure in elderly cardiac patients?

- Increased shortness of breath
- Greater fatigue
- Persistent coughing or wheezing
- Increased chest discomfort
- Difficulty sleeping
- Inability to lie flat
- Increased swelling in ankles and legs
- Sudden weight gain (within 2–3 days)
- Reduced physical activity
- Confusion or mental changes

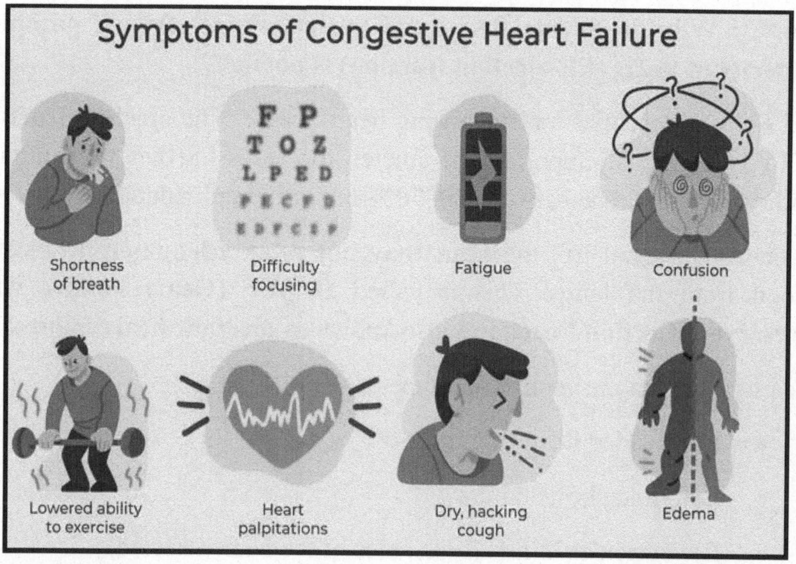

Q6.8.2: What tests are commonly advised when a cardiac patient presents with significant breathing difficulty?

Doctors assess the patient with clinical examination and the following investigations:

- **Chest X-ray** (and possibly CT chest if X-ray is abnormal)
- **ABG (Arterial Blood Gas Analysis)** – to assess oxygen and carbon dioxide levels
- **NT-ProBNP** (N-terminal pro-B-type natriuretic peptide) a blood test to help diagnose heart failure
- **ECG (Electrocardiogram)**
- **2D Echo (Echocardiography)**
- **Lung Ultrasound**
- **Routine blood tests**: CBP (Complete Blood Picture), RFT (Renal Function Test), etc.

Q6.8.3: Why do doctors use word 'heart failure' even if pumping capacity of heart (EF-ejection fraction) is normal?

2D Echo is essential for diagnosing heart failure. The **ejection fraction (EF)** is the most important parameter for assessing heart's pumping ability. EF should be between **50–70%** in normal individuals.

Even with normal EF, the heart **may not relax adequately** to receive blood from the lungs. This is called **HFpEF (Heart Failure with Preserved Ejection Fraction**), also known as **diastolic heart failure.**

Heart failure may have different types:

- Right-sided heart failure
- Left-sided heart failure
- Biventricular failure (both sides of the heart affected)

In patients with **extremely high blood pressure** (>180–200 mmHg), the heart struggles to pump against elevated resistance, causing **hypertensive heart failure**.

Hence one should know the exact cause of heart failure. It can be poor pumping capacity, poor relaxing capacity or extreme high blood pressure.

Q6.8.4: What is 'acute decompensation' in a patient with chronic heart failure?

- **Acute**: Recent and sudden onset
- **Chronic**: Long-standing condition (weeks to months)

Patients with chronic heart failure require consistent medication to prevent fluid overload and high blood pressure. If medication is missed or the patient develops another illness or infection, symptoms may worsen—this is referred to as **acute decompensation** or **ADHF (Acute Decompensated Heart Failure).** Such patients may come to ICU with breathlessness or swelling in legs and face. ICU admission is often required for these patients.

Q6.8.5: What treatment is available for heart failure?

Patients with heart failure need stabilization in ICU which can be achieved by following interventions:

- **Diuretic injections**: Such injections cause increased urine production to reduce fluid overload
- **NIV (Non-Invasive Ventilation)**: Provides oxygen support with pressure which helps to keep the lungs dry in case they are flooded with extra fluid due to congestion.
- **Medications to control the heart rate**
- **Medications to enhance cardiac pumping**
- **Medications to maintain adequate blood pressure**
- **Positioning**: Keeping patient upright to ease breathing

Once the patient is stabilized with above described interventions, they may need further cardiac monitoring for another **2–3 days**. All such cardiac patients need long-term medication for heart failure. Since there is **no permanent cure**, hospitalizations may occur frequently. **Heart transplantation** is the only curative treatment for specific type of heart failure and it is not suitable for every patient.

Q6.8.6: Why do some heart failure patients develop kidney failure too?

All organs require adequate blood flow. In heart failure, poor pumping may cause **low blood pressure**, affecting kidney and liver function. This condition is termed as **cardio-renal syndrome**. (means kidney functions are affected by reduced heart function)

Kidney failure may be **temporary** or **permanent** (depending on cardiac function and underlying conditions). Some patients may require **dialysis support** during ICU stay if kidney functions are hampered significantly.

Q6.8.7: Why do heart failure patients accumulate fluid around the heart or lungs?

This fluid is called an effusion:

Pericardial Effusion [fluid accumulation around the heart]: Pericardial effusion may result from fluid leakage due to poor heart pumping. If it impairs cardiac function, doctors may perform **pericardiocentesis**

(procedure to drain pericardial effusion in which small catheter is inserted in a cavity around the heart)

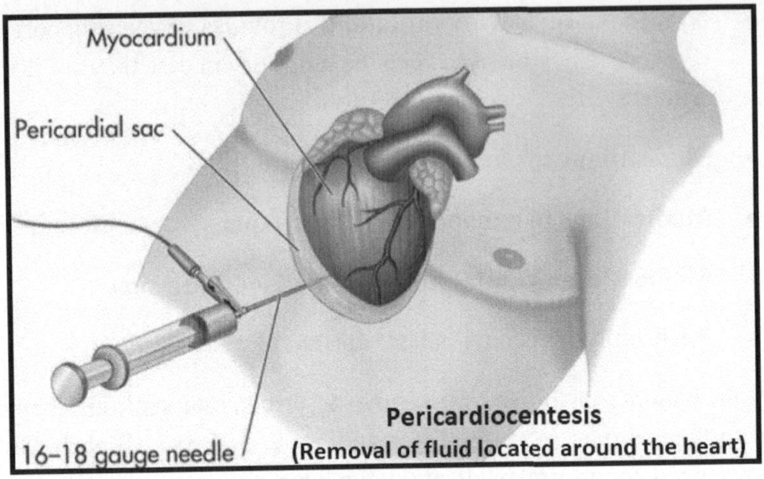

Pleural Effusion [fluid accumulation around the lungs]: Pleural effusion occurs when pressure builds in lung vessels, forcing fluid into the pleural cavity. If such fluid is causing any breathing difficulty or inadequate expansion of lungs, patient may need **pleurocentesis** (procedure to drain fluid which is accumulated around the lung with help of external tube insertion)

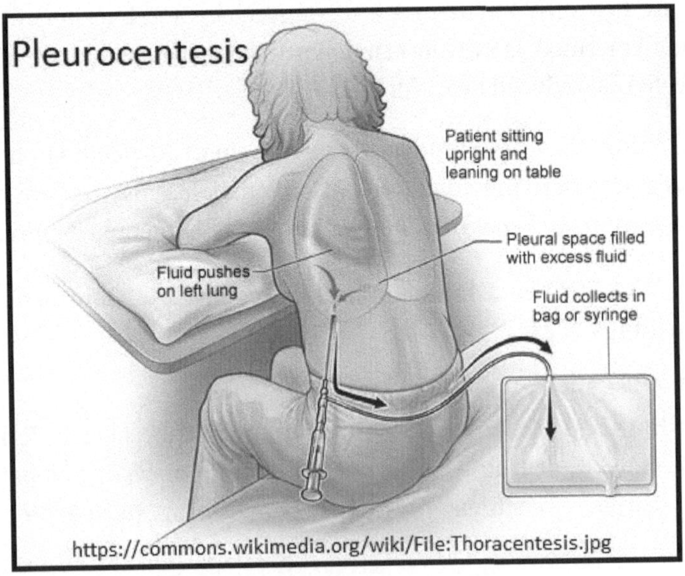

Q6.8.8: Why do patients with heart failure experience arrhythmias (heart rhythm disturbances)?

Heart failure causes **structural changes**—like chamber enlargement, wall thickening, or thinning—affecting electrical conduction and rhythm. Doctors may use different words to describe abnormal rhythm and it is better for patient's relatives to be familiar with such medical words.

Common arrhythmias (heart rhythm disturbances) include:

- **AF (Atrial Fibrillation):** very fast irregular heart rate
- **Atrial Flutter**
- **VT (Ventricular Tachycardia)**
- **SVT (Supraventricular Tachycardia)**
- **VF (Ventricular Fibrillation)**
- **Bradycardia:** very low heart rate
- **Various types of Heart Block:** extreme low heart rate

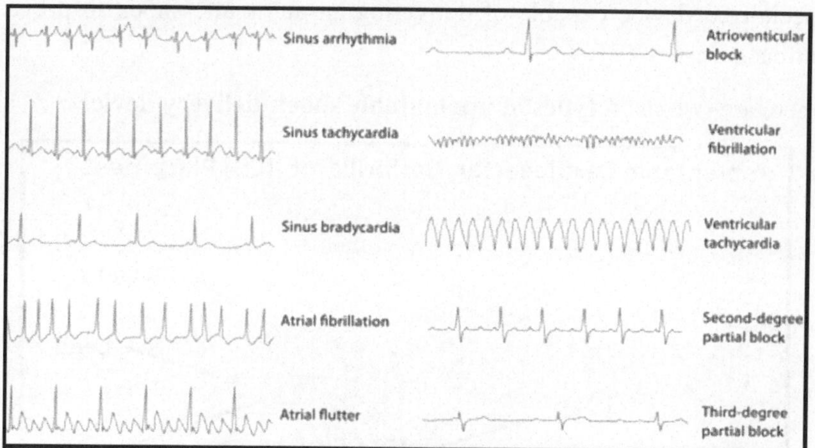

Different type of arrythmias

Some arrhythmias may lead to **cardiac arrest** (condition in which heart stops pumping blood adequately to all the organs and patient becomes unconscious and unresponsive because of abrupt cessation of blood supply to brain)

Treatment includes:

- **CPR (Cardiopulmonary Resuscitation)**
- **DC Shock** (Direct Current Shock) via defibrillator to restore rhythm
- **Anti-arrhythmic drugs**
- **Treating underlying cause** which is responsible for arrhythmia
- **Placement of Pacemaker** (for extreme low heart rate)

Q6.8.9: Why do some cardiac patients need permanent implantable battery-operated devices?

Patients with **extremely low heart rate** (bradycardia or heart block) may require an external electrical device to maintain a regular heartbeat. In such cases, **Permanent Pacemaker Implantation (PPI)** is advised.

When patients develop **sudden fatal arrhythmias** such as **ventricular tachycardia (VT)** or **ventricular fibrillation (VF)**, they may need a specialized device capable of delivering an automatic shock to prevent cardiac arrest.

There are **two** main **types of implantable shock-delivery devices**:

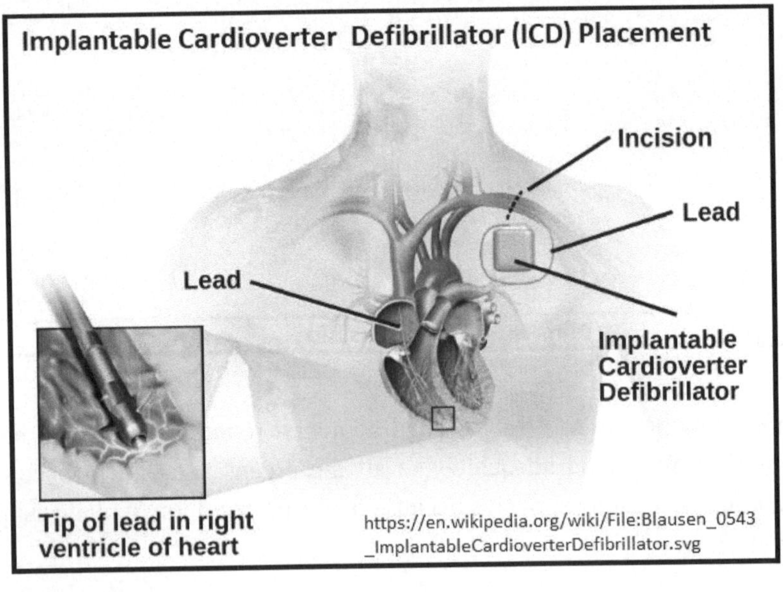

1. **ICD (Implantable Cardioverter Defibrillator)**
   a. Implanted in the chest under the skin
   b. Monitors heart rhythm continuously
   c. Delivers shock automatically upon detecting a dangerous rhythm
   d. Suitable for patients prone to arrhythmias—even without signs of heart failure

2. **CRT-D (Cardiac Resynchronization Therapy–Defibrillator)**
   a. Improves heart function and synchronizes heart chamber contractions
   b. Detects abnormal rhythms and delivers corrective shocks
   c. Enhances heart performance and overall quality of life

Diagnosis: 6.9 Chronic Liver Disease (CLD)

The **liver** performs vital functions including detoxification, bile production, energy storage, and regulation of blood clotting. **Chronic Liver Disease** refers to long-term damage, which may lead to **scarring (cirrhosis)** and eventually **liver failure**.

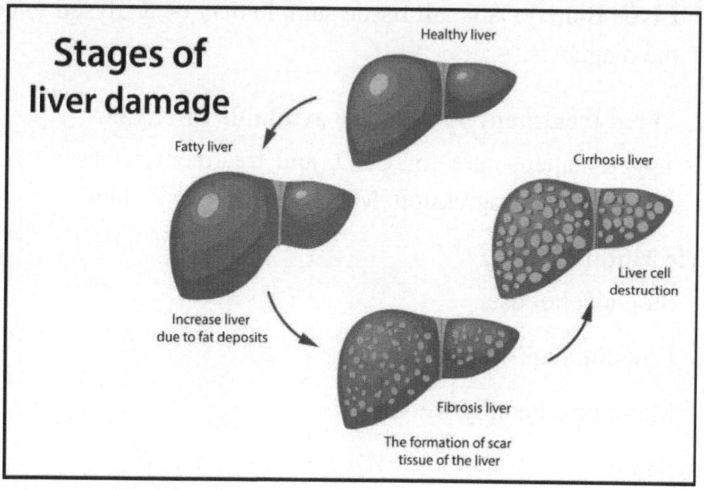

Common Causes of CLD:

- Long-term alcohol use
- Hepatitis infection

- Fatty liver disease
- Iron overload
- Copper deposition in liver
- Chemical/toxin exposure (e.g., vinyl chloride)

Symptoms of CLD:

- **Jaundice** (yellow discoloration of skin and eyes)
- **Abdominal pain or swelling** (due to fluid accumulation)
- **Dark urine, pale stools**
- **Fatigue and loss of appetite**
- **Unexplained weight loss**

Q6.9.1: How is chronic liver disease diagnosed?

Doctors rely on symptoms, physical exams, and the following tests:

- **Blood Tests**: Liver function tests (LFT) including bilirubin, albumin, and liver enzymes
- **Imaging**: Ultrasound, CT scan, and MRI of the abdomen
- **Liver Biopsy**: A small tissue sample may be analysed to confirm the diagnosis

Q6.9.2: What treatment options are available for CLD?

There's no permanent cure for CLD, and treatment is based on cause, severity, and disease progression. Management may include:

Lifestyle Modifications:

- Stop alcohol use
- Low-fat, high-fibre diet
- Maintain a healthy weight

Medications:

- **Diuretics** (medicines which helps in producing more urine)
- **Laxatives** (stool softener liquids or medications)
- **Antioxidants and multivitamins**

- **Immunosuppressants** (for autoimmune liver disease)
- **Antiviral drugs** (for hepatitis)
- **Antibiotics** (for infections)

Surgical/Procedural Options:

- **Liver transplant** (not suitable for all patients)
- **TIPS (Trans jugular intrahepatic portosystemic shunt) procedure**: By placing a stent to reduce excessive pressure in blood vessels of liver
- **Endoscopic ligation or sclerotherapy**: To stop bleeding from varices (swollen veins in the food pipe near the stomach)

Q6.9.3: Which liver functions are most affected in CLD?

- **Detoxification**: Inability to clear ammonia and toxins
- **Blood Clotting**: Reduced clotting factor production, increasing bleeding risk
- **Digestion**: Bile production decreases, causing indigestion
- **Blood Sugar Control**: Reduced glucose storage
- **Protein Production**: Low albumin levels cause body swelling
- **Immunity**: Weakened immune response increases infection risk

Q6.9.4: What complications may require hospitalization for the patients with CLD?

- **Ascites**: Fluid accumulation in the abdomen; may need **paracentesis** (ascitic tapping-removal of excessive fluid from abdominal cavity)
- **Cirrhosis**: Liver shrinks due to scarring which hampers important liver functions.
- **Variceal Bleeding**: Vomiting blood due to burst veins in the oesophagus
- **Jaundice**: Due to bilirubin build-up

- **Hepatic Encephalopathy**: Brain dysfunction from high ammonia; may cause irritability, sleep disturbance, or coma
- **Hepatorenal Syndrome**: Kidney failure due to liver dysfunction; few patients may require **dialysis** too

Q6.9.5: What is Spontaneous Bacterial Peritonitis (SBP) - a common problem in patients with CLD?

SBP is an infection of the **peritoneum** (membrane lining the abdomen) without any obvious tear or injury.

CLD patients often have **ascites** (fluid build-up in abdominal cavity), which can become infected if gut bacteria leak into the peritoneal cavity due to:

- Weakened immunity
- Changes in gut flora
- Increased intestinal permeability

Patients may present with **fever, chills, and abdominal pain**. Doctors may confirm SBP by analysing a fluid sample from ascites. Treatment involves **antibiotics**, ICU care, and possibly **dialysis** if kidney function worsens.

Q6.9.6: Who can be a donor for liver transplantation?

There are two types of liver donors:

a. **Living Donor:** A close relative (spouse, parent, sibling, or child aged 18–55 years) with a compatible blood type.
b. **Cadaveric Donor:** A person declared **brain-dead**—typically from severe head injury—whose heart continues to beat.

Note: Liver donation is not possible once the heart stops completely.

Q6.9.7: Why do some patients' relatives opt for 'end-of-life care' in chronic liver disease (CLD)?

There is no permanent cure for CLD other than **liver transplantation**, and many patients are not fit for such high-risk surgery.

If CLD progresses to brain involvement, patients may become unconscious and require ventilator support. Additionally, if kidney function deteriorates, dialysis may be needed—resulting in MODS (**multiple organ dysfunction syndrome)**. This worsens the prognosis significantly.

In cases where the patient is a **chronic alcoholic** and now needs intensive life support, families may choose **end-of-life care** to prevent further suffering from a disease that has **no definitive cure**.

Q6.9.8: What is 'decompensated chronic liver disease'?

CLD is considered **compensated** if the patient does not require hospitalization and continues regular daily activities. Such patients may not look or feel severely ill despite having advanced liver scarring.

When the **body can no longer cope**, CLD transitions to **decompensated status**, presenting with:

- **Jaundice** (yellowing of eyes and skin)
- **Ascites** (abdominal fluid causing distension and breathlessness)
- **Encephalopathy** (mental status changes such as drowsiness or irritability)
- **Variceal bleeding** (vomiting blood due to ruptured veins in the lower food pipe)

Patients with **decompensated CLD** often need **ICU admission**. Some improve with treatment, but many deteriorate and develop **MODS (Multiple Organ Dysfunction Syndrome)**—a critical condition with poor prognosis, often leading to death despite medical interventions.

Q6.9.9: Why do some CLD patients need a TIPS procedure?

TIPS (Trans jugular Intrahepatic Portosystemic Shunt) is performed by an interventional radiologist who places a **stent** in the liver to **reduce portal hypertension** (excess pressure in liver veins).

In CLD, the liver becomes resistant to blood flow, increasing pressure in vessels from the oesophagus, stomach, and intestines. This can lead to **variceal bleeding** (rupture of swollen veins) and **ascites** (abdominal fluid build-up)

TIPS procedure helps **redirect blood flow**, relieving pressure and reducing bleeding risk and ascites.

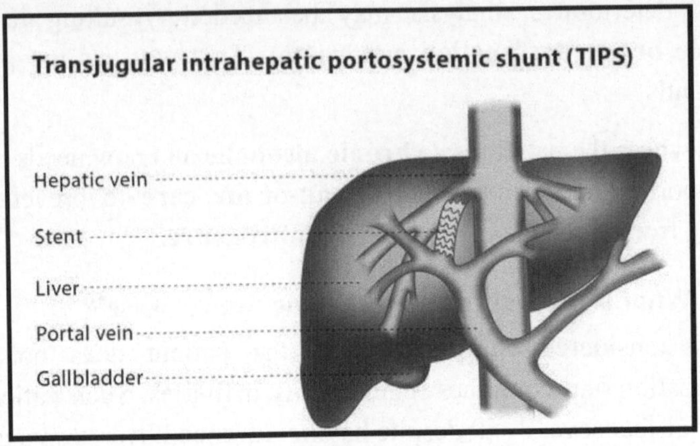

It may be recommended for:

- **Repeated variceal bleeding episodes**
- **Refractory ascites**
- **Liver transplant candidates awaiting donation**

Complications from TIPS can include:

- **Hepatic encephalopathy** (impaired mental status)
- **Infection**
- **Bleeding**

Q6.9.10: Why do patients with CLD remain malnourished despite appropriate treatment?

CLD patients—especially those with cirrhosis—often experience **progressive malnutrition** due to impaired digestion and nutrient absorption.

Causes include:

- Reduced bile flow, leading to poor fat absorption
- Loss of appetite
- Decreased energy intake
- Malabsorption in the gut

- Altered metabolism
- Hormonal disturbances
- Hypermetabolism
- Gut microflora imbalance
- Chronic inflammation
- Recurrent infections

These factors collectively compromise nutritional status, leading to **weight loss** and **muscle wasting** despite supportive care.

Diagnosis: 6.10 Pancreatitis

Pancreatitis is the inflammation of the pancreas; a vital organ located behind the stomach. The pancreas plays a key role in digestion by producing enzymes, and it regulates blood sugar through hormone production. Doctors may use the term **Acute Pancreatitis** for sudden onset and **Chronic Pancreatitis** for long-standing disease of pancreas.

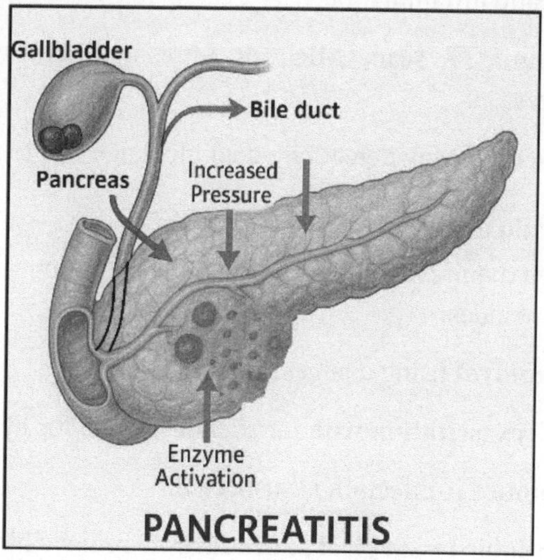

Q6.10.1: What are the causes of Pancreatitis?

Common causes include:

- **Gallstones**: These can block the bile duct and trigger inflammation.

- **Excessive alcohol consumption**: Heavy drinking inflames the pancreas.
- **Hypertriglyceridemia**: Elevated levels of triglycerides in the blood.
- **Medications**: Certain drugs like estrogen, steroids, and thiazide diuretics.
- **Infections**: Viral or bacterial infections.
- **Trauma or Surgery**: Physical injury or post-operative complications.

If no specific cause is identified, the condition is called **Idiopathic Pancreatitis**.

Q6.10.2: How is Pancreatitis diagnosed?

Diagnosis involves clinical symptoms and specific tests:

- **Blood Tests**: Elevated **amylase** and **lipase** enzymes indicate pancreatic inflammation.
- **Imaging**: CT scan, MRI, or ultrasound helps visualize the pancreas.
- **Endoscopy**: May detect bile duct blockage due to gallstones.

Q6.10.3: How do doctors treat Pancreatitis?

Treatment often requires **ICU admission** if the condition worsens quickly. Management includes:

- **Pain control** using analgesics.
- **Fluid resuscitation** with intravenous saline for hydration.
- **Antibiotics** if infection is suspected.
- **Endoscopic or surgical procedures** to remove blockages or dead tissue.
- Placement of **central and arterial lines** if blood pressure is critically low.

- **Ventilator support** for respiratory failure, and **dialysis** if kidneys are affected.

Q6.10.4: What complications can occur in Pancreatitis?

- **Pancreatic necrosis**: Death of tissue that may become infected.
- **Pancreatic pseudocysts**: Fluid-filled sacs requiring drainage if infected.
- **Diabetes**: Resulting from damage to insulin-producing cells.
- **Breathing difficulties**: May lead to respiratory failure.
- **Severe infections**: Can cause **septic shock**.
- **Organ failure**: May involve kidneys or liver.

Q6.10.5: When can the patient resume eating?

- Most patients are advised to **avoid food initially** due to nausea and pain.
- Early feeding (within **24–48 hours**) is encouraged once vitals stabilize.
- In severe cases, **tube feeding** that bypasses the stomach may be used to rest the pancreas.
- Feeding is delayed if the patient has **unstable blood pressure** or **severe illness.**

Q6.10.6: How can Pancreatitis be prevented?

While not all cases are preventable, risk can be reduced by:

- Avoiding **alcohol**
- Managing **body weight** to prevent gallstones
- Reducing **fat intake** in the diet
- Stopping **smoking**

Q6.10.7: How long do patients with Pancreatitis need to be in hospital?

Patients without complications typically recover in **4–7 days**. Those with severe pancreatitis and complications (e.g. septic shock) may need:

- **Prolonged ICU stay (2–3 weeks)**
- **Dialysis** for kidney failure
- **Ventilator support** for breathing difficulty

Q6.10.8: What is percutaneous drainage?

When fluid accumulates around the pancreas a **small catheter** is inserted under **ultrasound guidance** by an **interventional radiologist**.

- The procedure is **minimally invasive**—a simple needle puncture through the skin.
- It helps relieve pressure and reduce symptoms.

Q6.10.9: What surgeries may be required in severe cases of Pancreatitis?

When medications are not sufficient and complications arise:

- **Surgical debridement**: Removal of unhealthy tissue
- **Necrosectomy**: Removal of dead pancreatic tissue
- **Pancreatectomy**: Complete removal of the pancreas

These are **high-risk surgeries** with high mortality, and families should understand their seriousness.

Q6.10.10: What is ERCP (Endoscopic Retrograde Cholangiopancreatography) is and its role in pancreatitis management?

ERCP (Endoscopic Retrograde Cholangiopancreatography) is used when gallstones obstruct bile flow. ERCP is performed by a **medical gastroenterologist** under anaesthesia.

An **endoscope** is inserted through the mouth to visualize the bile and pancreatic ducts. It allows direct treatment of:

- **Stones**
- **Strictures** (narrow ducts)
- **Pseudocysts** (fluid filled cavities)

In comparison, **MRCP (Magnetic Resonance Cholangio-pancreatography)** is a **non-invasive MRI-based test** that helps visualize ducts and fluid collections. Some patients may undergo **MRCP** followed by **ERCP**, depending on the severity and cause of pancreatitis.

Diagnosis: 6.11 Cholecystitis

The medical term **"chole"** means bile, which is produced in the liver but stored in the **gallbladder**. Cholecystitis is an inflammation of the gallbladder. If gallstones form in the gallbladder, they can obstruct bile flow, leading to the accumulation of bile and bacterial infection. This type of infection is known as **acute cholecystitis** (acute means 'new onset' or developed very recently).

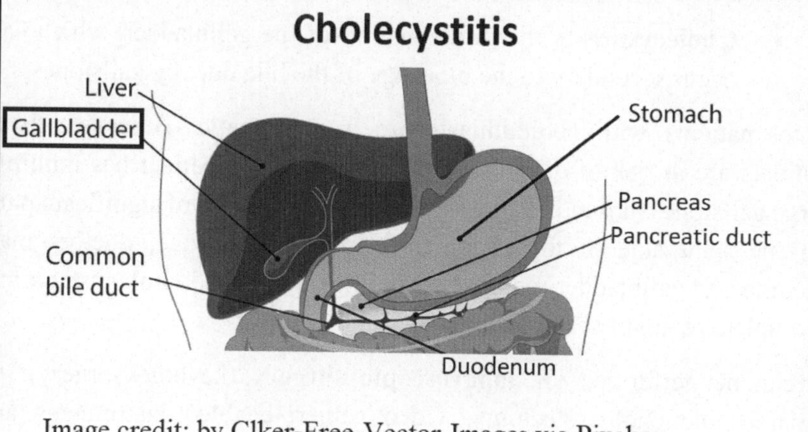

Image credit: by Clker-Free-Vector-Images via Pixabay

Apart from gallstones, other factors can also cause cholecystitis. If a patient develops cholecystitis without the presence of gallstones, it is referred to as **acalculous cholecystitis**. This type can occur due to trauma, severe illness, prolonged fasting, or severe infection. Critically ill patients with acalculous cholecystitis may have multiple complications due to the complex nature of their condition.

Q6.11.1: How do doctors diagnose cholecystitis?

In addition to clinical findings such as **pain** on the right side below the rib cage, **fever**, **nausea**, and **vomiting**, certain blood tests and radiological investigations help diagnose cholecystitis.

- Blood tests may show elevated white blood cell counts and abnormal liver function.
- Ultrasound and CT scan of the abdomen can provide more accurate information about gallbladder infection and other major abdominal abnormalities.

Diagnosis is made based on the patient's symptoms, blood test results, and imaging findings.

Q6.11.2: What is the difference between cholecystitis and cholelithiasis?

- **Cholelithiasis** refers to the presence of multiple gallstones in the gallbladder.
- **Cholecystitis** is the inflammation of the gallbladder, which can occur secondary to the blockage of the bile duct by gallstones.

Most patients with cholelithiasis are asymptomatic. However, these patients are at risk of developing cholecystitis. If a patient has multiple large gallstones (around 10 mm) with repeated episodes of significant pain on the right side of the abdomen below the rib cage, doctors may recommend gallbladder removal. This surgery is called **cholecystectomy** (complete removal of the gallbladder).

It can be performed via **laparoscopic surgery** (keyhole surgery). In laparoscopic cholecystectomy, video camera-enabled instruments are inserted through small incisions in the abdomen. This technique helps avoid major scars. Patients who are not fit for laparoscopic surgery may require an **open cholecystectomy**, where the surgeon makes a larger incision (cut over the skin) to remove the gallbladder.

Q6.11.3: What treatment is provided to patients with cholecystitis in the ICU?

Some patients with cholecystitis may require invasive procedures or surgery, while others may improve with conservative treatment.

Conservative treatment includes:

- Antibiotics
- Intravenous fluids
- Pain relief medications
- Nutritional support
- Hydration and correction of electrolyte imbalances

If a patient is not stable enough for surgery, the doctor may recommend a **percutaneous cholecystostomy**—an invasive procedure where a drainage tube is placed in the gallbladder to relieve distension by draining pus or bile.

If the patient is stable, **laparoscopic** or **open cholecystectomy** (operation to remove gallbladder) can be performed—often within 72 hours of diagnosis. In critically ill patients, surgery may be postponed until the condition improves.

Q6.11.4: Why is acalculous cholecystitis considered more dangerous than calculous cholecystitis?

Acalculous cholecystitis typically arises as a complication of serious illness, infection, or injury that damages the gallbladder. It is more common in critically ill patients suffering from **sepsis** or other conditions requiring ICU admission. Such patients may need prolonged antibiotic therapy and are at risk of major complications, including:

- **Perforation of the gallbladder** (rupture due to excessive fluid accumulation)
- **Necrosis** (extensive tissue damage due to cell death)

Calculous cholecystitis, on the other hand, is often manageable through surgery, provided the patient is stable. In some cases, a drainage procedure may be needed before surgery. These patients are usually more stable at diagnosis and better tolerate complications.

Q6.11.5: What complications can occur in patients with cholecystitis?

- **Gangrene** or **necrosis of the gallbladder**: Severe infection may lead to tissue death, requiring urgent surgical removal.
- **Perforation**: The gallbladder may rupture, causing **peritonitis** (infection of the abdominal lining) or **abscess** (localized pus collection).
- **Sepsis and septic shock**: Despite appropriate antibiotics, infection may progress to septic shock—a life-threatening drop in blood pressure.
- **Bile duct injury**: This may occur during surgical intervention.

Q6.11.6: Can a patient live a normal life after gallbladder removal surgery (cholecystectomy)?

- Yes, a person can live perfectly well without a gallbladder. There are usually no long-term effects after gallbladder removal.
- Some patients may need **digestive enzyme supplements** (lipase, protease, amylase) and **vitamins**.
- If a patient experiences diarrhoea or bloating, doctors may prescribe medications and advise avoiding fatty foods such as fried items. Since fat digestion becomes difficult for many, it's also recommended to avoid late-night meals.

Diagnosis: 6.12 Urosepsis with Acute Kidney Injury

The urinary tract is the body's drainage system for removing urine. It includes two kidneys, two ureters, a bladder, and a urethra. An infection in any of these organs is known as a **urinary tract infection (UTI)**, which can spread to the bloodstream, leading to a severe and potentially life-threatening condition called **urosepsis**.

- **Cystitis**: Infection of the urinary bladder
- **Pyelonephritis**: Infection of the kidneys

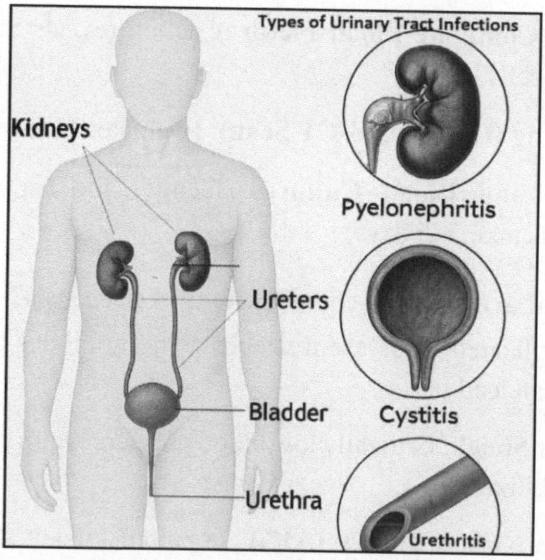

Some patients present with severe UTI that progresses to **septic shock** (significantly low blood pressure due to infection). Low blood pressure and dehydration can impair kidney function, resulting in elevated **creatinine levels**. A normal creatinine level in blood is below 1.35 mg/dL. Elevated levels suggest **AKI (acute kidney injury-** sudden rise in creatinine levels because of dehydration, low blood pressure or any other reasons), which may take days to weeks to resolve.

Patients with urosepsis may have symptoms like:

- High-grade fever and chills
- Groin pain
- Painful and frequent urination
- Rapid breathing and elevated heart rate

Initial treatment includes antibiotics, intravenous fluids, and supportive care. Few patients may require surgery to control the source of infection.

Q6.12.1: How is a diagnosis of UTI and urosepsis made?

Along with clinical symptoms, specific investigations are used:

- **CUE (Complete Urine Examination)**: May show pus cells in urine

- **CBP (Complete Blood Picture)**: Often reveals increased white blood cells
- **Imaging (Ultrasound/CT Scan)**: Evaluates kidneys and bladder
- **Urine and Blood Cultures**: Identify the causative bacteria (results take 3–5 days)

Q6.12.2: What are possible complications of urosepsis?

While uncomplicated UTIs are treatable with antibiotics and hydration, severe cases can lead to:

- **Septic Shock**: Critically low blood pressure requiring medications to stabilize
- **Acute Kidney Injury (AKI)**: Impaired kidney function due to infection, obstruction, or reduced blood flow
- **Multi-Organ Dysfunction Syndrome (MODS)**: If toxins accumulate, it may affect brain, lungs, heart, and liver. Patients may require ventilator and dialysis support

Q6.12.3: Why is urine catheterization advised for some patients?

Urine catheterization involves placing a **Foley's catheter** into the bladder via the urethra. It's used to monitor urine output accurately, especially in patients with:

- Elevated creatinine
- Low blood pressure
- Altered consciousness
- Post-surgery or prolonged bed rest

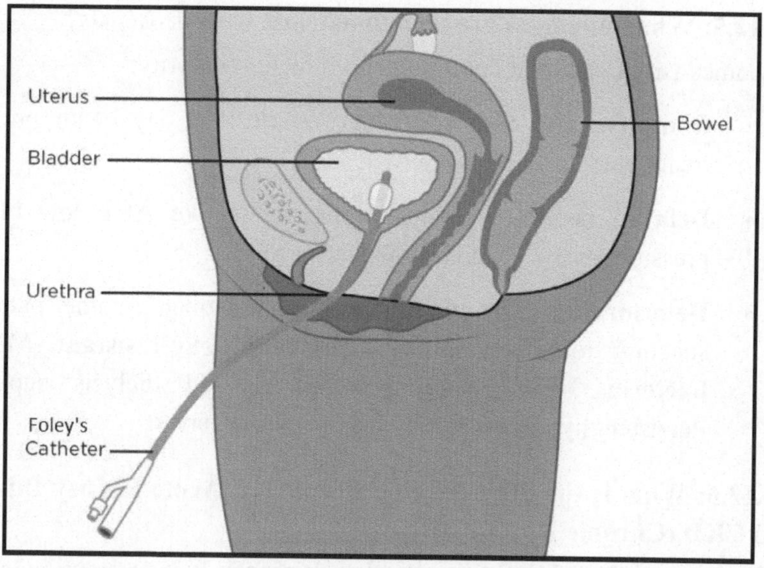

Hourly measurement helps guide fluid and medication management. Catheters also help avoid skin contamination in bed-bound patients.

Q6.12.4: When is surgery necessary for complicated UTIs?

Antibiotics alone may not suffice if:

- Pus or fluid accumulation needs drainage
- Urine flow is obstructed, causing **hydroureteronephrosis** (urine build-up and kidney swelling)

Surgical options include:

- **DJ Stenting**: A tube placed between kidney and bladder to allow drainage
- **Percutaneous Nephrostomy (PCN)**: Drain tube inserted directly into kidney
- **Nephrectomy**: Removal of infected kidney in **emphysematous pyelonephritis**
- **Cystoscopy**: Camera-assisted bladder inspection if catheters repeatedly get blocked
- **Suprapubic Catheter (SPC)**: Tube inserted into bladder through the lower abdomen when urethral access is impossible

Q6.12.5: What outcomes are seen in patients with urosepsis?

Outcomes vary by patient condition and infection severity:

- **Complete and fast recovery**: Within 4–5 days with prompt treatment
- **Delayed recovery**: With complications like AKI, low blood pressure, or the need for dialysis/surgery
- **Deterioration and death**: Despite treatment, some patients succumb to infections caused by **multidrug-resistant (MDR) bacteria**, often requiring ventilator and dialysis support. Persistent hypotension may lead to cardiac arrest

Q6.12.6: What is the difference between AKI (Acute Kidney Injury) and CKD (Chronic Kidney Disease)?

AKI (Acute Kidney Injury) is a **sudden** decline in kidney function, often triggered by an event like infection, dehydration, low blood pressure or blood loss, and is typically reversible with treatment. Kidney size remains normal in patients with AKI.

CKD (Chronic Kidney Disease) is a **gradual**, progressive loss of kidney function over months or years, often due to conditions like diabetes or high blood pressure, and is generally not reversible. Kidney size often found reduced (smaller sized kidneys) in patients with CKD.

Q6.12.7: Is lifelong dialysis required after ICU dialysis initiation?

Not necessarily. Dialysis may be temporary for patients with **AKI** due to an acute illness. If the illness resolves and kidney function recovers, dialysis can be discontinued.

However, patients with **CKD**, especially with advanced damage from diabetes or hypertension, may need **long-term dialysis** due to **irreversible** loss of kidney function.

Q6.12.8: What are different types of dialysis commonly practiced in ICU?

Patients with CKD who are dialysis dependent may require dialysis twice or thrice a week, and they do not need admission to ICU for such regular dialysis sessions. Such kind of regular dialysis is considered as **IHD**

(Intermittent Haemodialysis), which can be provided to patients in a day-care facility because it takes only 3–4 hours to complete one dialysis session.

IHD (Intermittent Haemodialysis) is a type of dialysis that can also be used for patients who are getting treated in ICU if they don't have extremely low blood pressure. This type of dialysis can cause a further drop in blood pressure immediately after initiating the dialysis session in few ICU patients.

If a patient has significantly low blood pressure, doctors may advise another type of dialysis that does not cause a significant drop in blood pressure. **SLED (Sustained Low-Efficiency Dialysis)** is a type of dialysis that is advised for patients with low blood pressure to avoid sudden drop and change in blood pressure, as SLED is continued for a longer duration (6 to 8 hours) with a low blood flow rate. The same dialysis machine can be used for SLED, which is generally used for IHD.

Extremely sick patients in ICU who are requiring multiple medicines to increase or support the blood pressure may benefit from **CRRT (Continuous Renal Replacement Therapy)**. CRRT is a type of dialysis that runs continuously without any interruption and requires a special dialysis machine (CRRT machine).

Sometimes doctors may advise **HDF (Hemodiafiltration)** for a few sick patients to avoid major fluctuations in blood pressure during the dialysis session. HDF is also a type of dialysis that can be extended for a longer duration (more than 12 hours if needed).

Q6.12.9: What is AV fistula (Arteriovenous Fistula), and why do doctors advise AV fistula operation to patients with CKD (chronic kidney disease)?

If a patient requires dialysis support in ICU, dialysis is done through a haemodialysis sheath (a dialysis catheter placed near the neck, collarbone or groin area through which blood goes to the dialysis machine and returns to the body). This catheter can be used for a few weeks, but there are high chances of infection if the dialysis catheter is kept for a longer duration, hence doctors may advise permanent access for dialysis to patients who need dialysis regularly. Apart from a lower infection rate, there are other benefits of AV fistula compared to dialysis catheter as vascular access, like better blood flow, durability, and improved dialysis efficiency.

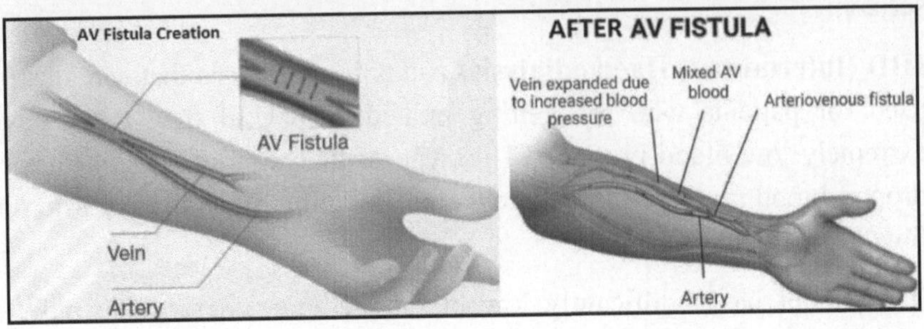

An AV fistula (Arteriovenous Fistula) is a surgically created permanent access for dialysis through which dialysis can be done regularly. Either a vascular surgeon or a cardiothoracic surgeon performs surgery on the arm to create a connection between an artery and a vein near the elbow joint. The vein becomes dilated and easily visible after a few weeks of surgery, and doctors may advise further dialysis sessions through the newly formed matured AV fistula. Till the AV fistula becomes functional, the patient may need HD sheath as vascular access for dialysis sessions.

Various complications can happen to patients with AV fistula. Bleeding from the fistula site, blood clot formation, and failed non-functional fistula are the most common complications seen in patients with AV fistula. A few patients may require another surgery to create another AV fistula if the first AV fistula becomes non-functional.

Q6.12.10: What are the possible complications that can happen during dialysis?

- Sudden drop in blood pressure
- Vascular access-related complications (bleeding, blood clot or fistula failure)
- Electrolyte imbalance (higher or lower levels of sodium, potassium and calcium)
- Muscle cramps
- Brain swelling (Dialysis Disequilibrium Syndrome: a very serious condition that occurs due to a rapid change in blood chemistry

causing neurological symptoms like confusion, nausea, headache or altered mental status)

- Cardiac rhythm disturbance (irregular heartbeats)
- Itching
- Shivering

Diagnosis: 6.13 Skin and Soft Tissue Infections (SSTIs)

Skin and soft tissue infections (SSTIs) are frequently encountered infections in ICU where the skin and deeper structures are involved. These infections are very common in elderly patients, as they have low immunity and they are prone to various infections. Just like any other organ of the body, skin is an important part which can easily become an entry point for infection, and such infection can also involve deeper structures below the skin (fat tissues and muscles).

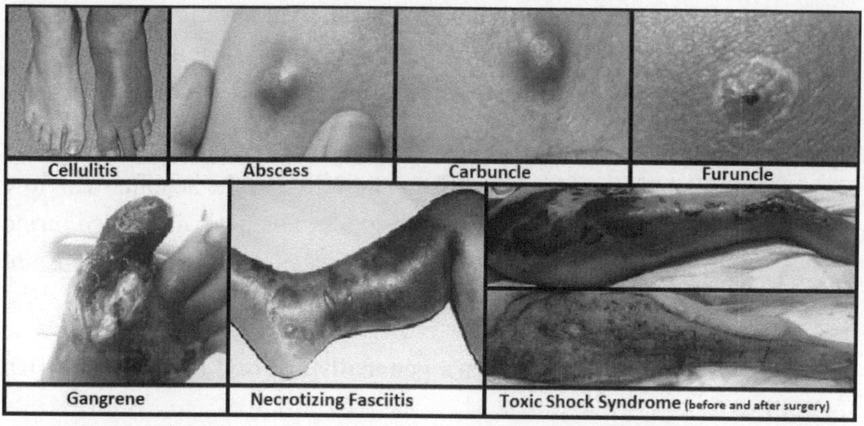

Examples of SSTIs:

Cellulitis (diffuse infection of the skin and underlying tissue which makes the skin red, swollen and painful)

Abscess (painful and pus-containing swelling beneath the skin which can appear initially as a boil)

Carbuncle (painful and large swelling over the skin which occurs if multiple boils merge and create a cluster of boils)

Furuncle (infection of hair follicle which appears as a painful and pus-filled swelling over the skin)

Gangrene (dead tissue due to severe infection or loss of blood supply to the tissue)

Necrotizing fasciitis (very serious skin and soft tissue infection which involves multiple layers between skin and muscles)

Toxic shock syndrome (very serious disease caused by bacterial toxins leading to fever, skin rashes and extremely low blood pressure)

Q6.13.1: Why do patients with cellulitis need admission in ICU?

- Cellulitis may appear as a minor skin infection initially, but it can spread to adjacent tissues rapidly and the patient may deteriorate faster if appropriate treatment is delayed.
- Patients may have excessive pain and swelling over the affected limb, for which continuous pain-relief medications are needed. Such medications are given through an infusion pump, which requires constant monitoring too. Hence, patients may need to be treated in ICU even if their vitals are stable.
- Some patients with cellulitis get admitted to the hospital with low blood pressure, constant high-grade fever or decreased urine output. Such patients must be treated in ICU for constant monitoring to prevent further deterioration.

Q6.13.2: What investigations are generally advised for patients with cellulitis?

All patients admitted to ICU may need blood investigations (complete blood picture, creatinine, C-reactive protein, electrolytes), but patients with cellulitis may need ultrasonography of the affected limbs to assess the extent of infection.

Some patients whose legs are swollen may need a "**lower limb venous Doppler test**," which is done by a radiologist. This test is done to rule out **DVT** (deep vein thrombosis: presence of blood clots in deep veins of the legs), which can also cause pain and swelling in the legs.

Q6.13.3: Why is surgery required for some patients with cellulitis?

Most patients with cellulitis get better with intravenous antibiotics. Hydration with intravenous fluids and dressing with magnesium sulphate can be advised to patients with cellulitis, but some patients may not show faster recovery if the infection has involved deeper structures or extensive areas. If swelling is significant, it can compress the blood vessels causing poor blood supply to the distal part of the limb. To prevent such a complication, it is necessary to reduce the pressure over the blood vessels caused by swelling. A surgical incision can release the tension under the skin, and such surgical intervention is known as "**fasciotomy**" (an incision or cut through the skin, muscle and fascia — a thin covering surrounding the muscles).

Sometimes pus is seen under the skin, and it must be removed by a minor surgical procedure known as **"I and D" (incision and drainage)**, in which the surgeon gives a small nick on the infected area to drain the pus out.

Q6.13.4: What kind of complications can occur in patients with cellulitis?

Just like any other infections, cellulitis too can cause multiple complications despite appropriate treatment.

- **Acute kidney injury (AKI):** Kidney functions may be affected by severe infections (particularly if infection causes profound low blood pressure), and some patients may need dialysis support if the kidneys are affected significantly
- **Compartment syndrome:** If swelling in the legs or arms causes extreme pressure on the tissue and blood vessels, the surgeon must intervene to release the pressure
- **Gangrene:** Extensive tissue damage and death of tissue, requiring amputation
- **Sepsis:** When infection spreads to other parts of the body through the blood, causing low blood pressure, the patient's clinical condition may deteriorate further

Diagnosis: 6.14 Gastroenteritis

Gastroenteritis is an inflammation or infection of the stomach and intestines, and it is usually caused by viruses, bacteria or parasites. Undercooked food or contaminated water can also cause Gastroenteritis.

Patients may show symptoms like nausea, vomiting, diarrhoea, stomach cramps or fever. If a patient cannot drink or eat adequately, dehydration can occur easily because of ongoing loss of fluid and electrolytes through vomiting and loose stools. The major treatment is fluid therapy and electrolyte replacement.

Q6.14.1: Why do patients with gastroenteritis need admission in ICU?

Most patients with gastroenteritis do not require hospitalization. But if patients are losing excessive fluid through vomiting and loose stools, they may show symptoms like lethargy, giddiness or decreased urine output. Such patients may need hospitalization for fluid therapy and close monitoring.

Despite appropriate treatment, many patients continue to have loose stools for a longer duration if the infection is severe, and doctors can replace the fluid and electrolytes immediately if patients are being treated in ICU. Some electrolyte imbalances can affect heartbeats, hence constant monitoring of heart rate and blood pressure is essential, which is only possible in ICU.

Patients with severe dehydration may come to the hospital with reduced urine output, and they may need dialysis support if urine output does not improve with fluid therapy. Initiation of dialysis must be done in ICU for such patients, and hence ICU admission is a must for all patients with severe gastroenteritis.

Q6.14.2: Why do some patients have persistent diarrhoea even after initiation of treatment?

Diarrhoea (loose stools) may persist for hours to days despite appropriate treatment. If the infection is severe, it may take a longer duration for relief from diarrhoea.

Many patients suddenly develop diarrhoea after staying in the hospital for a longer duration because of prolonged antibiotic exposure.

Sometimes patients may have persistent diarrhoea because of viral or parasitic infection, as antibiotics mostly help in bacterial diarrhoea.

Some chronic inflammatory conditions can be responsible for persistent diarrhoea, for which specific treatment is required for long-term management.

Q6.14.3: What kind of tests may doctors advise for patients with gastroenteritis?

- **Blood tests:** complete blood picture, renal function test along with electrolytes, liver function test, blood culture
- **Stool tests:** stool routine examination, stool for ova and parasite examination, stool culture
- **Radiological tests:** X-ray or CT scan of the abdomen (not always)
- **Ultrasound:** ultrasonography of the abdomen
- **Endoscopy and colonoscopy:** to observe the internal structure of the stomach and intestines (not required for all patients with gastroenteritis)

Q6.14.4: How long is treatment needed for gastroenteritis?

If patients with gastroenteritis are admitted to ICU, they may need a minimum of 3 to 4 days of ICU stay for fluid and electrolyte replacement along with continuous monitoring of urine output.

Some patients who develop complications like acute kidney injury (elevated creatinine level or reduced hourly urine output) may need a longer ICU stay until their kidney function improves. It may take a few days to a few weeks for complete recovery of kidney function if the kidneys sustain significant insult due to dehydration.

Some patients may continue to have adequate urine output despite elevated creatinine and urea levels. Such patients may not need dialysis support if their creatinine levels decrease gradually after initiation of treatment. If

AKI (acute kidney injury) resolves faster, patients may have a shorter stay (less than a week) in ICU.

Q6.14.5: Why do some patients require sigmoidoscopy or colonoscopy if they have persistent loose stools?

Colonoscopy is a procedure to see the internal lumen of the large intestine (colon), and sigmoidoscopy is a procedure to examine the lower part of the colon. Some patients with gastroenteritis may have continuous diarrhoea for a longer duration despite appropriate antimicrobial therapy and other measures. Such patients need to be evaluated further for the exact cause behind persistent diarrhoea. A medical gastroenterologist is the specialist who performs colonoscopy and sigmoidoscopy to examine the internal lumen of the colon with the help of a colonoscope.

Apart from infective causes, there are other clinical conditions in which prolonged diarrhoea can happen. Inflammatory bowel disease, colon cancer or polyps (abnormal growth inside the colon) can also cause persistent loose stools, and colonoscopy is a very important diagnostic procedure to detect these medical conditions.

Q6.14.6: What are the possible complications found in patients with severe gastroenteritis?

- Severe dehydration
- Severe electrolyte imbalance (change in sodium or potassium levels)
- Acute kidney injury (few patients may need dialysis too)
- Weight loss and malnutrition
- Haemolytic uremic syndrome (kidney failure and red blood cell destruction can happen in some patients with gastroenteritis)
- Reactive arthritis (**very rare** complication in which joints get affected after gastroenteritis)
- Guillain-Barré Syndrome (GBS) [**extremely rare** condition in which a patient develops weakness in limbs a few weeks after gastroenteritis]

Chapter - 7

Conversations in ICU Counselling Room

When a loved one is critically ill, the counselling room becomes a space where families seek clarity, reassurance, and difficult truths. For many, it's the first time they hear terms like "ventilator support," "dialysis," or "end-of-life care"—often delivered in moments of emotional vulnerability.

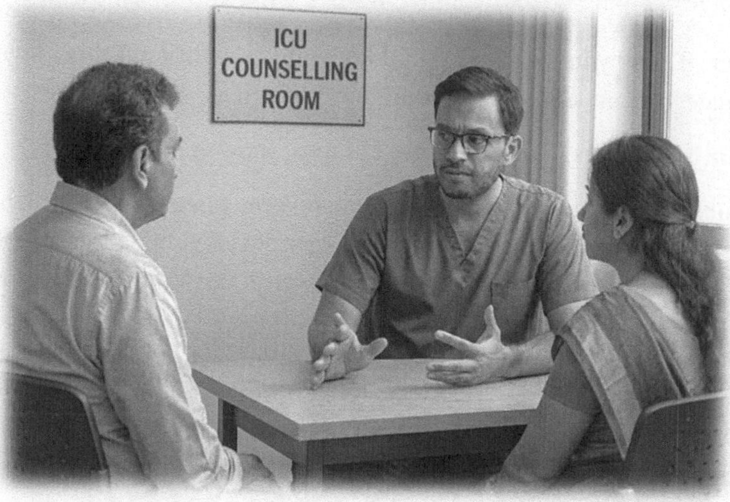

This chapter presents real-life examples of conversations between ICU doctors and patients' relatives, designed to help families feel more familiar with the language, tone, and emotional weight of these discussions.

Each scenario reflects the delicate balance intensivists must maintain: offering medical facts with compassion, guiding decisions with honesty, and respecting cultural and emotional contexts. By understanding how these conversations unfold, readers can better prepare themselves to ask questions, absorb information, and participate meaningfully in their loved one's care.

7.1: Conversation about ventilator support

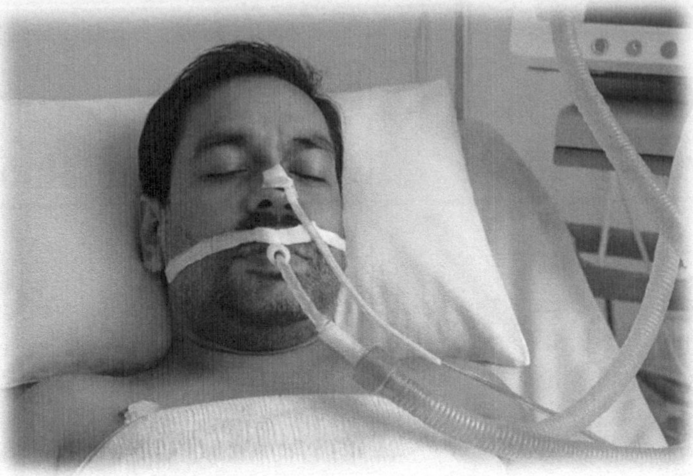

Doctor: Thank you for coming in. I know this is a difficult time. I wanted to update you on your father's condition and discuss the next steps.

Patient's son: Yes, Doctor. Please tell me… how is he doing now?

Doctor: Your father has developed **severe pneumonia**, which has significantly affected his lungs. His oxygen levels dropped despite high-flow oxygen, so we had to place him on a ventilator to support his breathing.

Patient's son: Ventilator means life support, right? Is it very serious?

Doctor: Yes, being on a ventilator means he needs full support for breathing. It is a serious condition, but this support gives us a chance to treat the infection and improve his condition. Without this support, it would have been very difficult for him to survive.

Patient's son: How long will he need to be on the ventilator?

Doctor: It is difficult to predict right now. Some patients improve in a few days, but for some it can take longer. We will try to remove the ventilator support as soon as his lungs are strong enough to work on their own.

Patient's son: Is there a risk to his life?

Doctor: I want to be honest with you. Yes, severe pneumonia requiring ventilator support does carry a **significant risk**, especially in critically ill patients. But please remember, we are doing everything possible with all available ICU facilities to give him the best chance of recovery.

Patient's son: Is he in pain? Can he hear us?

Doctor: He is sedated for comfort, so he is not in pain. While deeply sedated, he may not be fully aware, but we encourage family members to speak to him—sometimes familiar voices can be reassuring.

Patient's son: What are you doing to treat the infection?

Doctor: He is on strong intravenous antibiotics, and we are monitoring his vitals closely. We have also started supportive care—fluids, nutrition, and medications to maintain blood pressure and prevent complications.

Patient's son: Is there anything we should do?

Doctor: Right now, being present is important.

Patient's son: We'll do that. My mother wants to do a small prayer near his bed. Is that okay?

Doctor: Absolutely. We will make sure she has a quiet moment with him. We will keep you informed daily. If there's any change—good or bad—you'll be the first to know.

Patient's son: Thank you, Doctor. I just hope he pulls through.

Doctor: We are doing everything we can. Let's take it one day at a time.

7.2: Conversation about dialysis support

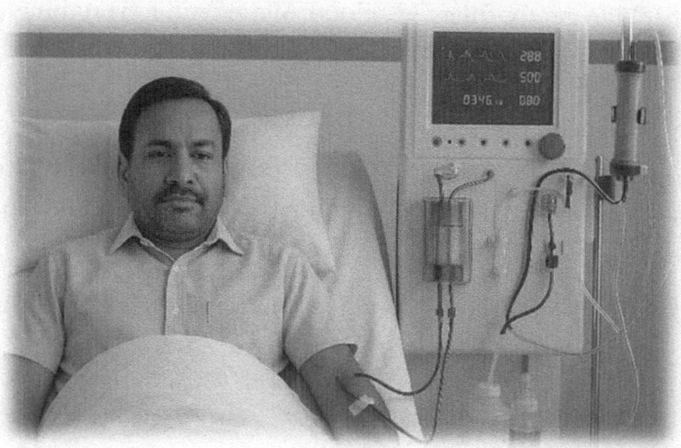

Doctor: Thank you for coming in. I wanted to update you on your husband's condition and discuss an important step in his treatment.

Patient's wife: Yes, doctor. He has been unconscious since yesterday. The nurse said his urine output is very low. What's happening?

Doctor: Your husband came in with severe sepsis—an overwhelming infection that affected multiple organs. One of the major complications has been a drop in blood pressure, which reduced blood flow to his kidneys. As a result, his kidney function has deteriorated significantly.

Patient's wife: So his kidneys are failing?

Doctor: They're not working well right now. His body is not clearing toxins or excess fluid, and his potassium levels are rising, which can affect the heart. To support him, we recommend starting dialysis—specifically, a gentle form called **continuous renal replacement therapy** or **CRRT**, which is suitable for ICU patients.

Patient's wife: Will dialysis cure his kidneys?

Doctor: Dialysis doesn't cure the kidneys—it supports them while we treat the underlying infection. In some cases, kidney function can recover once the sepsis improves. But right now, dialysis is essential to prevent further complications and give his body a chance to heal.

Patient's wife: Is it painful? Will he feel anything?

Doctor: He is sedated and he is on a ventilator, so he won't feel discomfort. We insert a dialysis catheter—usually in the neck or thigh—and the machine gently filters his blood. We monitor everything closely.

Patient's wife: Are there risks?

Doctor: Like any procedure, there are risks—bleeding, infection at the catheter site, or blood pressure changes. But in his case, the risks of not doing dialysis are far greater. Without it, toxins will build up and his condition may worsen rapidly.

Patient's wife: He is a strong man. He fought through diabetes and heart issues. I just want to do what's best.

Doctor: And you are. This decision is about giving him the best possible support. We will keep you informed every step of the way. If you are comfortable, we will begin dialysis today once you give consent.

Patient's wife: Yes, doctor. Please go ahead. And… thank you for explaining everything so clearly.

Doctor: You are most welcome. We are here with you, every step.

7.3: Conversation about ICU procedures

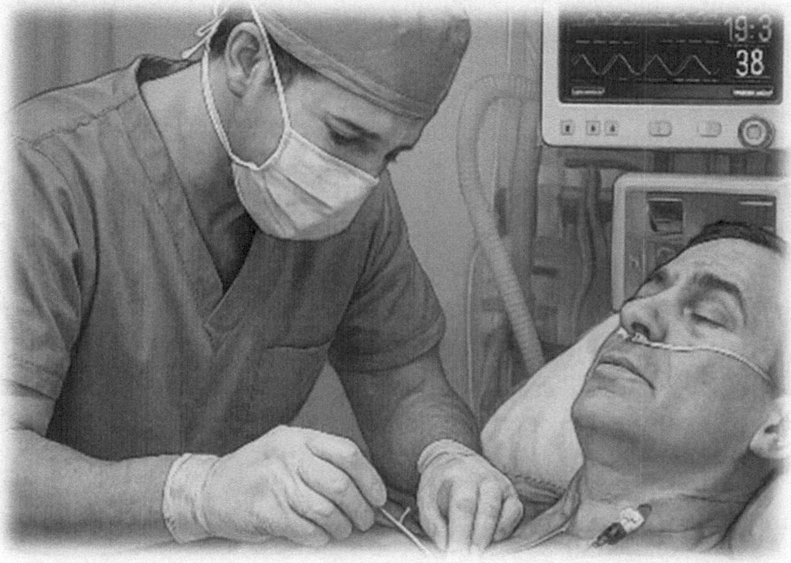

Doctor: I want to give update about your son's condition.

Patient's mother: What about his blood pressure now?

Doctor: His blood pressure is dangerously low, a condition we call **shock**. This means his organs are not getting enough blood flow and oxygen to function properly. We have been giving him fluids and medications to try to raise it, but we need to do more to get an accurate picture of what's happening and to administer stronger medication more effectively.

Patient's mother: What do you mean by "more"?

Doctor: To manage his blood pressure and give him the best chance of recovery, we need to insert two special lines: a **central line** and an **arterial**

line. I want to explain what they are and why they are so important right now.

Patient's mother: Are they tubes? Is this an operation?

Doctor: They are sterile tubes, yes, but they are not major surgery. They are bedside procedures we perform right here in the ICU. The **arterial line** is a very small catheter, like an IV, that we place into an artery, usually in his wrist. This gives us a continuous, moment-by-moment reading of his blood pressure. The monitors you see now only give us a reading every few minutes, but with an arterial line, we will know instantly how he is responding to treatments. This helps us make immediate adjustments to his medication doses.

Patient's mother: Okay, I understand that. What about the other one?

Doctor: The **central line** is a slightly larger catheter that we place into a large vein, usually in his neck or chest. This line is crucial for two main reasons. First, it allows us to give him the powerful medications needed to support his blood pressure. These medications are too strong for a regular IV (intravenous) in the hand or arm and can damage smaller veins. The central line ensures the medication gets to his heart quickly and safely. Second, it allows us to draw blood for lab tests without having to poke him multiple times a day.

Patient's mother: So, are these risky?

Doctor: They are very common procedures in the ICU. As with any procedure, there are small risks, such as bleeding or infection, but we take every precaution to minimize them. To be honest, the risk of not placing these lines is far greater. They are absolutely essential for us to provide the level of care he needs right now. We need these tools to stabilize him and give his body a chance to fight.

Patient's mother: So you are saying we can't save him without them?

Doctor: We can't provide the precise, real-time care he needs without them. This is the next critical step. These procedures will allow us to monitor him more accurately and to administer the life-saving medication he requires to get his blood pressure up and keep his organs working. Our top priority is to stabilize him, and these lines are a fundamental part of that plan.

Patient's mother: Okay. If you think it's what he needs, then we trust you.

Doctor: Thank you. We will proceed once you give written consent and we will update you about his condition again within few hours.

7.4: Conversation about Angiogram (coronary angiography)

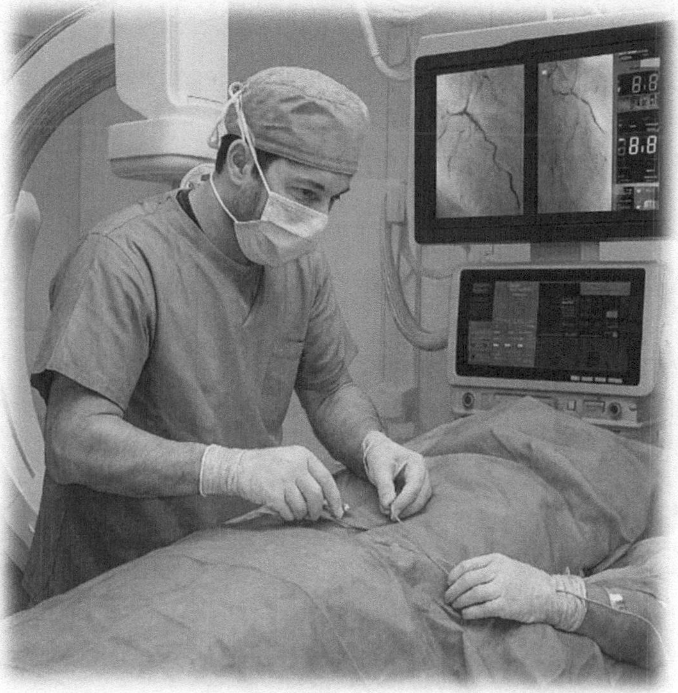

Doctor: Thank you for coming in. I would like to update you on your father's condition and discuss the next steps.

Patient's son: Doctor, we are worried. You said he was improving, but now he is back on the ventilator again?

Doctor: Yes, he was stable enough for a trial off the ventilator, but each time we tried, he developed fluid in the lungs—what we call **pulmonary**

edema. This makes breathing extremely difficult and forces us to re-intubate (initiating invasive ventilator support again).

Patient's son: Why is this happening again and again?

Doctor: We suspect the underlying cause may be related to his heart. Specifically, poor blood flow to the heart muscle—what we call **ischemia**—can lead to weak pumping and fluid buildup in the lungs. This could explain the recurrent pulmonary edema.

Patient's son: So what do you recommend?

Doctor: We need to perform a coronary angiography. It's a procedure where we inject dye into the heart's blood vessels and take detailed images to see if there are any blockages.

Patient's son: Is it safe to do this while he's on the ventilator?

Doctor: It's not without risk, but we'll take all precautions. The procedure is done in a specialized Cath-lab (cardiac lab), and he will be closely monitored throughout. The information we get could be life-saving and it will guide us on whether he needs stenting, medications, or other interventions.

Patient's son: If we don't do it?

Doctor: We will be treating blindly. Without knowing the state of his coronary arteries, we can't address the root cause. He may continue to have fluid overload and remain ventilator-dependent.

Patient's son: We understand. Please go ahead. Just… keep us informed.

Doctor: Of course. We will arrange for the angiography as soon as possible and update you immediately after. You are doing the right thing.

7.5: Conversation about emergency surgery

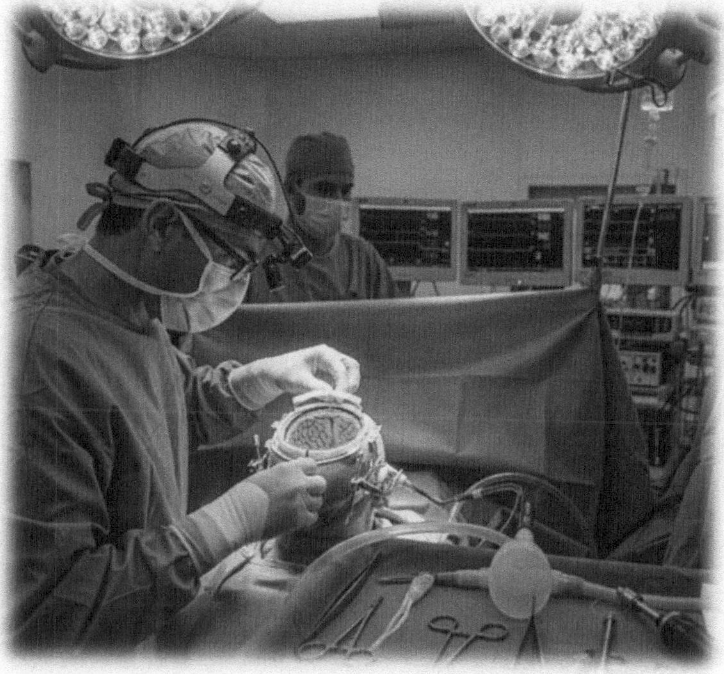

Neurosurgeon: Thank you for coming in quickly. I need to speak with you about your husband's condition. There's been a sudden and serious change.

Patient's wife: Doctor, he was talking to me just this morning. What happened?

Neurosurgeon: Yes, when he arrived, his GCS (Glasgow Coma Scale) was normal. But over the past few hours, he has become increasingly drowsy and now he is not responding to verbal commands. We repeated the brain scan, and it shows a large **subdural hematoma**—bleeding between the brain and its outer covering.

Patient's wife: Is that why he is not waking up?

Neurosurgeon: Exactly. The blood is putting pressure on his brain, causing swelling and shifting of brain structures. This is life-threatening.

If we don't act immediately, it could lead to irreversible brain damage or death.

Patient's wife: What can be done?

Neurosurgeon: We need to take him for emergency neurosurgery—specifically, a **craniotomy**. We will open a part of the skull, evacuate the clot, and relieve the pressure. The sooner we do this, the better his chances of survival and recovery.

Patient's wife: Is it risky?

Neurosurgeon: Any brain surgery carries risks—bleeding, infection, seizures—but in this case, not doing the surgery is far more dangerous. Time is critical. Every minute of delay increases the risk of permanent damage.

Patient's wife: Will he be the same after surgery?

Neurosurgeon: It's hard to predict. Some patients recover well, especially if surgery is done early. Others may have weakness, speech issues, or memory problems. But right now, our goal is to save his life and prevent further deterioration.

Patient's wife: We understand. Please do whatever is needed.

Neurosurgeon: Thank you. We will take him to the operating theatre immediately. I will update you as soon as the procedure is done.

7.6: Conversation about 'end-of-life' care

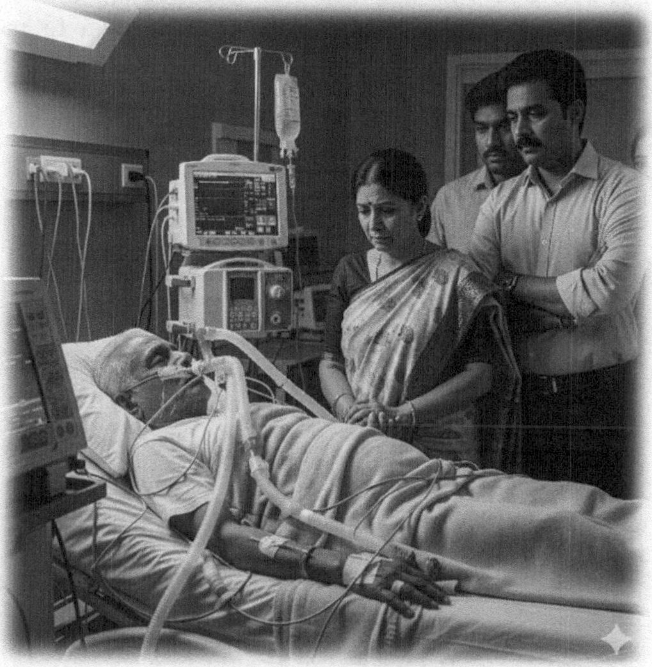

Relative: Doctor, how is my father now?

Doctor: I know this is very difficult. Your father had a major stroke and later a cardiac arrest. Even though his heart was revived, his brain has suffered severe and permanent damage. He is not expected to recover or wake up.

Relative: But he is on the ventilator… is that keeping him alive?

Doctor: Yes. The ventilator is doing the work of his lungs, and medicines are supporting his blood pressure. Without these machines, his body would not survive.

Relative: Does that mean he is suffering?

Doctor: Continuing these machines may only prolong his suffering, without any chance of meaningful recovery. In such situations, we often discuss **end-of-life care** — focusing on comfort and dignity instead of machines and procedures.

Relative: What is end-of-life care?

Doctor: It means stopping treatments that no longer help, like the ventilator or strong medicines, and instead giving medicines to keep him peaceful, pain-free, and comfortable. This allows him to pass away naturally, with dignity.

Relative: That sounds very hard… but we don't want him to suffer.

Doctor: I understand. This is a very tough decision. We will fully support you and ensure he does not feel pain or distress.

Relative: Can we have some time to talk as a family?

Doctor: Of course. Take the time you need. I will be here to answer any questions. And when you are ready, we will proceed with documentation of "end-of-life" care.

Chapter - 8

What To Do And What Not To Do?

When a loved one is admitted to the ICU, family members often encounter a hospital environment that feels unfamiliar and overwhelming. Sometimes, due to lack of awareness about ICU rules and protocols, relatives may unintentionally make mistakes during their visit. Such unintentional actions can potentially impact the patient's clinical condition. If patients and their families are informed about basic ICU guidelines and procedures in advance, they can navigate the ICU setting with greater confidence.

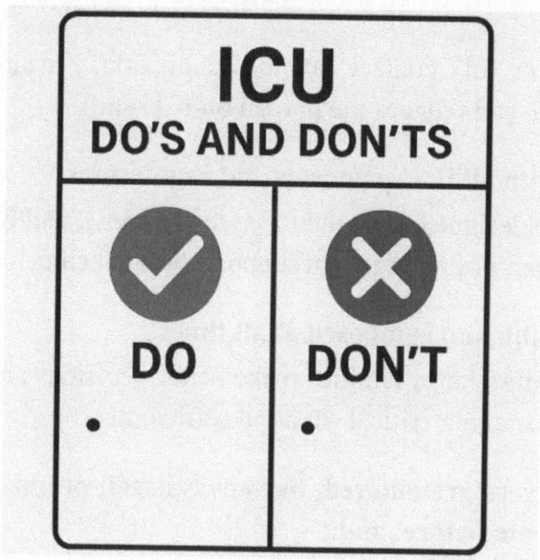

It is important to understand what actions are inappropriate or discouraged within the ICU. Even without intending harm, a relative's behaviour may interfere with the patient's recovery. Therefore, it is essential to know both the recommended and discouraged practices when someone is admitted to the ICU.

8.1: Do's for Patient's Relatives

1. **Always sanitize your hands with antiseptic solution or hand sanitizer before and after touching the patient.**

ICU patients are highly vulnerable to infections. Proper hand hygiene prevents transmission of harmful microbes and protects both the patient and healthcare staff.

2. **Adhere strictly to the designated ICU visiting hours.**

Visiting hours are structured to balance patient rest, medical procedures, and family interaction. Respecting them ensures smoother care delivery.

3. **Share the patient's complete medical history and previous medical records when requested by the medical team.**

Accurate and timely information helps doctors make informed decisions, especially in emergencies or when complications arise.

4. **Designate one family member as the primary contact for receiving updates.**

A single point of contact avoids confusion, ensures consistent communication, and reduces the burden on ICU staff.

5. **Comply with all ICU protocols and regulations.**

These rules are designed to maintain safety, hygiene, and order in a high-risk environment. Following them supports optimal care.

6. **Remain calm and composed at all times.**

Emotional stability helps families make better decisions and supports the ICU team in managing critical situations efficiently.

7. **Quiet prayers are allowed, but always seek permission from the medical team beforehand.**

Spiritual support is valuable, but it must be practiced in a way that doesn't interfere with medical care or disturb other patients.

8. Speak gently with ICU staff, even if the patient's condition is extremely serious.

Respectful communication fosters trust and collaboration between families and healthcare providers.

9. Ask questions in a respectful manner.

Clarifying doubts is important, but tone and timing matter. Courteous inquiries encourage open dialogue.

10. Uphold the patient's dignity throughout the stay.

Treating the patient with respect—regardless of their condition—preserves their humanity and emotional well-being.

11. Avoid loud or dramatic expressions of grief.

Such reactions can distress other families and disrupt the calm environment needed for patient recovery.

12. Request simple explanations if medical terminology is difficult to understand.

Doctors are willing to simplify complex terms. Asking for clarity ensures informed consent and better understanding.

13. Limit the number of visitors while the patient is in the ICU.

Fewer visitors reduce infection risk and allow the patient to rest without unnecessary stimulation.

14. Maintain a notebook or diary to record important updates.

Keeping track of medical information helps families stay organized and reduces repeated queries to staff.

15. Try to communicate with the patient during visiting hours, even if they are semiconscious or unconscious.

Familiar voices can offer emotional comfort and may positively influence recovery, even if the patient cannot respond.

16. **Inquire about possible complications before giving consent for any ICU procedures.**

Understanding risks helps families make informed decisions and prepares them for potential outcomes.

17. **Be patient while waiting for medical documents such as investigation reports, summaries for second opinions, discharge papers, or death certificates.**

These documents require careful preparation and verification. Patience ensures accuracy and avoids unnecessary pressure on staff.

8.2: Don't's for Patient's Relatives

1. **Avoid carrying mobile phones into the ICU; if permitted, keep them on silent mode.**

Phones can interfere with sensitive equipment and disturb the quiet ICU environment. Silence ensures safety and respect.

2. **Do not take photographs while inside the ICU.**

Photography violates patient privacy and hospital policy. It may also distract staff during critical care.

3. **Refrain from speaking loudly or disturbing other patients.**

Noise can cause stress and disrupt the healing process for all patients in the ICU.

4. **Do not use your phone loudly, even in the waiting area outside the ICU.**

Loud conversations can disturb others who are anxious or grieving. A quiet atmosphere is more respectful.

5. **Never touch any medical equipment.**

ICU devices are highly sensitive and essential for patient survival. Tampering can lead to serious consequences.

6. **Do not argue with the medical staff.**

Disputes can delay care and create unnecessary tension. Concerns should be raised calmly and through proper channels.

7. **Avoid overstaying during or beyond the designated visiting hours.**

Extended visits may interfere with medical routines and patient rest. Timely departure shows consideration.

8. **Do not request frequent updates; ICU doctors typically provide updates once or twice daily.**

Constant inquiries can overwhelm staff and distract from patient care. Scheduled updates ensure clarity and efficiency.

9. **Refrain from asking nurses about treatment plans or clinical decisions.**

Nurses follow doctors' instructions and may not be authorized to discuss medical strategies. Direct queries to the appropriate personnel.

10. **Do not display aggressive behaviour toward doctors or ICU staff, even if you disagree with their explanations.**

Aggression undermines trust and may compromise communication. Constructive dialogue is more effective.

11. **Do not overcrowd the ICU; limit visitors to a maximum of two at a time.**

Overcrowding increases infection risk and disrupts the controlled ICU environment. Limited access protects everyone.

12. **Do not bring outside food or medications for the patient without prior approval from the doctor.**

Unapproved items may conflict with treatment plans or pose health risks. Always consult the medical team first.

13. **Avoid public displays of extreme emotion such as loud crying or panic.**

While emotions are natural, intense reactions can unsettle other families and staff. Private spaces are better suited for grieving.

14. **Do not offer money or tips to housekeeping or ICU staff.**

Gratitude is appreciated, but monetary gestures may violate hospital ethics and policies.

15. Avoid seeking multiple opinions from different relatives, as this may lead to confusion during critical decision-making.

Unified decision-making prevents delays and miscommunication. Trusting the designated contact ensures clarity.

16. Don't visit if you're sick.

Anyone with a fever, flu-like symptoms, a cold, or any other signs of infection should not visit the ICU

Glossary

2D-ECHO: two-dimensional echocardiography (study of heart structure functions with the help of ultrasonography)

ABG: Arterial Blood Gas (blood test to check oxygen and carbon dioxide levels in the blood along with few other important components)

Abscess: localized pus collection

Acute: new onset or developed very recently

ADHF: Acute Decompensated Heart Failure (worsening of symptoms in patient with chronic heart failure)

AECOPD: Acute Exacerbation of COPD (Chronic Obstructive Pulmonary Disease)

AF: Atrial Fibrillation (very fast irregular heart rate)

AKI: Acute Kidney Injury (sudden rise in creatinine levels because of dehydration, low blood pressure or any other reasons)

Aneurysmal bleed: bleeding secondary to rupture of abnormal dilated blood vessel

Angioplasty: repair of blood vessels (by stent placement or balloon dilation)

Antiplatelet drugs: blood thinner drugs

Apnoea Test: a test to confirm brain-death (apnoea means absence of breathing)

Arousable: person who is sleepy but easily awakened

Arterial line: a line which can be inserted at the wrist or groin to monitor blood pressure continuously

Ascites: Fluid accumulation in the abdomen

Aspiration pneumonia: pneumonia secondary to aspiration (entry of saliva, secretions or stomach content into lungs), mainly occurs to semiconscious or unconscious patients

Ataxia: poor balance and difficulty in walking

Autonomic dysfunction: significant fluctuations in blood pressure, heart rate, or temperature

AV fistula: Arteriovenous Fistula (surgical creation of dialysis access for patients with chronic kidney disease)

BiPAP: Bilevel Positive Airway Pressure (type of non-invasive ventilation mode)

Blood vessels: tubes through which blood flows to organs

Bradycardia: very low heart rate

Brain-dead: Unconscious and unresponsive patient with absent brainstem functions like breathing, coughing or swallowing

Bulbar muscles: muscles in the mouth and throat that control speech and swallowing

CABG: Coronary Artery Bypass Graft (cardiac surgery to re-establish blood circulation to the cardiac muscles by bypassing the affected blood vessels using grafts)

CAG: Coronary angiogram (an invasive procedure to check blood flow through important vessels to the muscles of heart)

Carbuncle: painful and large swelling over the skin which occurs if multiple boils merge and create a cluster of boils

Cardiogenic Shock: persistently low blood pressure secondary to heart dysfunction

Cardio-renal syndrome: clinical condition in which kidney functions are affected by reduced heart function

CBP: Complete Blood Picture (to check haemoglobin, white blood cells and platelet counts)

Cellulitis: diffuse infection of the skin and underlying tissue which makes the skin red, swollen and painful

Central line: a line which can be inserted near the neck or collarbone to give multiple medicines at once

Cerebellum: part of brain which is responsible for balance and coordination

Chemotherapy: treatment of cancer patients with anticancer drugs

Cholecystectomy: complete removal of the gallbladder

Cholecystitis: inflammation of gallbladder

Cholelithiasis: presence of multiple gallstones in the gallbladder

CIP: critical illness polyneuropathy (extreme muscle weakness and nerve damage due to prolonged ICU stay)

Cirrhosis: scarring of liver which hampers important liver functions

CKD: Chronic Kidney Disease (long term kidney disease)

CLD: Chronic Liver Disease (long term illness because of liver dysfunction)

Coma: person who has no voluntary movement and who does not respond to stimuli

Contusion: head injury which can cause bruising in brain tissue

CPAP: Continuous Positive Airway Pressure (type of non-invasive ventilation mode)

CPR: Cardiopulmonary Resuscitation (life saving measure which includes chest compressions and breathing support to unresponsive person)

Cranioplasty: surgery to reattach the bone and repair the skull defect

CRRT: Continuous Renal Replacement Therapy (continuous dialysis support for extremely sick patients with very low blood pressure)

CRT-D: Cardiac Resynchronization Therapy–Defibrillator (device which can give shock automatically and also help improving cardiac function

CSF: Cerebrospinal Fluid (fluid present in the brain which is circulating around the brain tissue and spinal cord)

CTICU: Cardiothoracic ICU-where patients are kept after cardiac or thoracic surgeries

CUE: Complete Urine Examination (urine test)

CVC: Central Venous Catheter (central line to give medication directly near the heart)

Cystitis: infection of the urinary bladder

Cystoscopy: Camera-assisted bladder inspection if catheters repeatedly get blocked

Debridement: removal of unhealthy tissue

Decannulation: removal of any cannula or tube (example: tracheostomy tube removal)

Decompressive craniectomy: removal of a part of the skull bone to allow the brain to expand and relieve the pressure

Delirium: awake patient but confused, with abnormal behaviour

Diagnosis: identification of disease, condition or injury

Disoriented: person who does not recognize place or people

Drowsy: person who is very sleepy

DVT: Deep Vein Thrombosis (blood clot in leg veins due to poor mobility)

ECG: Electro Cardiogram (test that records the electrical activity of heart using electrodes placed on chest, arms, and legs)

ECMO: Extracorporeal Membrane Oxygenation (machine to support lungs and heart)

ECPR: Extracorporeal Cardiopulmonary Resuscitation (ECMO initiation during ongoing CPR)

EDH: Extradural Hematoma (blood collection outside the outer layer of the brain)

EEG: Electroencephalogram-a test to record electrical activity of brain (mainly for patients with altered conscious level)

EF: ejection fraction (pumping capacity of heart)

EOL care: end-of-life care (conservative and palliative care to the patients with terminal illness or extreme poor prognosis)

ERCP: Endoscopic Retrograde Cholangiopancreatography (diagnostic and therapeutic endoscopic procedure for patients with gallstone related obstruction of bile flow)

Fasciotomy: an incision or cut through the skin, muscle and fascia — a thin covering surrounding the muscles

FiO_2: Fraction of Inspired Oxygen (ventilator setting which decides how much oxygen is given to patient)

Furuncle: infection of hair follicle which appears as a painful and pus-filled swelling over the ski

Gangrene: dead tissue due to severe infection or loss of blood supply to the tissue

GCS: Glasgow Coma Scale (scoring system to assess consciousness)

Haemorrhagic conversion: if bleeding happens inside the ischemic stroke area of brain

Haemorrhagic stroke: bleeding in the brain

Hepatic Encephalopathy: Brain dysfunction secondary to high ammonia liver in patients with liver failure

Hepatorenal Syndrome: Kidney dysfunction or failure due to liver dysfunction

HFNC: High-Flow Nasal Cannula (special equipment to deliver very high amount of oxygen support)

HFpEF: Heart Failure with Preserved Ejection Fraction (when heart muscles can't relax adequately also known as diastolic heart failure)

HIE: Hypoxic Ischemic Encephalopathy (irreversible brain damage due to low oxygen reaching the brain)

HRCT Chest: High-Resolution Computed Tomography of chest (detailed CT scan of chest to assess lungs)

Hydrocephalus: accumulation of cerebrospinal fluid in the brain

Hyperosmolar therapy: use of specific injections to reduce the pressure in the skull

Hypertensive bleed: bleeding in the brain because of extreme high blood pressure

Hypertriglyceridemia: Elevated levels of triglycerides in the blood.

Hypoxemia: low blood oxygen level

I and D: incision and drainage (surgical procedure in which the surgeon gives a small nick on the infected area to drain the pus out)

IABP: Intra-Aortic Balloon Pump (special device to support the heart function during or after coronary intervention)

ICCU: Intensive Coronary Care Unit-where patients with heart attack or who needs stenting for coronary artery disease

ICD: Implantable Cardioverter Defibrillator (device which can detect heart rhythm disturbance and deliver shock automatically)

ICD: Intercostal Drain (a tube inserted through chest wall to remove air or fluid which is collected around the lung)

ICH: Intracranial Haemorrhage (bleeding in the skull cavity which can be in the brain or outside of brain tissue)

ICP: Intra-Cranial pressure (pressure in the skull)

ICU: Intensive Care Unit- where critically ill patients are being treated

Idiopathic: where exact reason is not identified for any medical condition

IHD: Intermittent Haemodialysis (regular dialysis)

Infusion pump: device to give intravenous medications at specific rate in which larger syringe can be kept to infuse accurate dose of medications during specific time-period

Intensivist: specialist doctor who treats and manages patients in ICU

Intubation: placement of a breathing tube into the windpipe

Ischemic stroke: blockage in blood vessels of the brain

IV: Intravenous (medications which are given through catheter into the vein)

Jaundice: yellow discoloration of skin and eyes

LAMA: Leave Against Medical Advice

Lazarus sign: a rare reflex found in brain dead patients which can cause sudden movement of limbs secondary to spinal reflexes

LFT: Liver Function Test (to check bilirubin, liver enzymes and albumin levels)

Locked-in State: Completely paralyzed but fully conscious patient

Malabsorption: poor absorption of nutritional substances from gut into the blood

MDR: multidrug-resistant (organisms which can't be killed by common antibiotics because of the resistance to multiple antibiotics)

Mechanical thrombectomy: a catheter-based procedure done in a Cath-lab by a specialist to remove the blood clot from affected blood vessel

Mechanical ventilation: breathing support with specific device like ventilator

MI: Myocardial Infarction (heart attack)

MICU: Medical ICU-where nor-surgical patients are being treated

Midbrain: central brain area involved in important functions like swallowing, coughing, and breathing

MODS: Multiple Organ Dysfunction Syndrome (extreme critical condition when more than 2 organs are affected)

MRCP: Magnetic Resonance Cholangio-pancreatography (it is a non-invasive MRI-based test that helps visualize ducts and fluid collections)

MRI: Magnetic Resonance Imaging- It is useful to identify abnormal findings in brain and other organs of the body by doing a scan with help of MRI machine (patient has to lie down without making any movements for few minutes during MRI scan)

NCSE: Non-Convulsive Status Epilepticus (continuous electrical discharges from the brain which is documented by EEG while patient might not show any visible seizure activity)

Necrosectomy: Removal of dead pancreatic tissue or other dead tissue

Necrosis: dead tissue

Necrotizing fasciitis: very serious skin and soft tissue infection which involves multiple layers between skin and muscle

Nephrectomy: removal of infected kidney

NICU: Neonatal ICU-where newborn children are getting treatment

NIV: Non-Invasive Ventilation mask (face mask to provide ventilator support without inserting tube in windpipe)

NT-ProBNP: N-terminal pro-B-type natriuretic peptide (a blood test to help diagnose heart failure)

Obtunded: person with moderate reduction in alertness

Pancreatectomy: complete removal of the pancreas

Pancreatic pseudocysts: Fluid-filled sacs around pancreas which may require drainage if infected.

Paracentesis: ascitic tapping (removal of excessive fluid from abdominal cavity)

PCI: Percutaneous Coronary Intervention (stent placement or balloon dilation for major blockages of blood vessels which supply blood to heart muscles)

PCN: Percutaneous Nephrostomy (surgical drain tube inserted directly into kidney to remove pus)

PEEP: Positive End-Expiratory Pressure (ventilator setting which helps to keep lungs inflated)

PEG: Percutaneous Endoscopic Gastrostomy- Invasive procedure in which feeding tube is placed by a medical gastroenterologist using an endoscope (tube enters the stomach through the skin of the abdomen)

Percutaneous: any procedure done through skin route

Perforation: rupture or small hole

Pericardiocentesis: procedure to drain pericardial effusion in which small catheter is inserted in a cavity around the heart

Peritonitis: infection of the abdominal lining

PICC: Peripherally Inserted Central Catheter (intravenous line which is placed near forearm but the tip of the catheter reaches near the heart)

PICU: Paediatric ICU-where kids of different ages are treated and monitored

Pleurocentesis: procedure to drain fluid which is accumulated around the lung with help of external tube insertion

Pneumothorax: Air leakage around lung

Portal hypertension: excess pressure in liver veins

PPI: Permanent Pacemaker Implantation (device which prevents extreme low heart rate)

Prognosis: the likely outcome of a disease or the chance of recovery

Provisional diagnosis: a tentative diagnosis made by doctors when they suspect a particular condition but need more information to be certain

PTCA: Percutaneous Transluminal Coronary Angioplasty (invasive procedure in which stent is placed in the coronary vessels to establish adequate blood flow)

PTE: Pulmonary Thromboembolism (obstructed blood flow to the lungs due to big blood clot formation in blood vessels carrying blood to lungs)

Pyelonephritis: infection of the kidneys

Re-intubation: inserting the breathing tube again if patient doesn't breathe adequately after removal of ventilator support

RFT: Renal Function Test (to check creatinine, electrolytes and urea levels)

RICU: Respiratory ICU-where patients with lung diseases are getting treated

Ryle's tube: feeding tube which is inserted through nostril or mouth which is also known as NG tube (nasogastric tube)

SAH: Subarachnoid Haemorrhage (diffuse bleeding in multiple areas of the brain)

SBP: Spontaneous Bacterial Peritonitis (infection of the membrane lining the abdomen without any obvious tear or injury)

SDH: Subdural Hematoma (blood collection under the outer layer of the brain)

Seizures: fits (uncontrolled movements of limbs due to abnormal electrical discharge that occurs within the brain)

Sepsis: severe infection for which patient requires ICU admission

Septic Cardiomyopathy: infection-related cardiac failure

Septic Shock: severe infection causing extreme low blood pressure

SICU: Surgical ICU-where patients are kept after surgery for post-operative monitoring

SLED: Sustained Low-Efficiency Dialysis (longer duration dialysis for critically ill patients)

SPC: Suprapubic Catheter (tube inserted into bladder through the lower abdomen when urethral access is impossible)

SSTIs: Skin and soft tissue infections

Statins: drugs to reduce cholesterol levels in the blood

Status epilepticus: continuous fits like activity

Stupor: person who is difficult to wake and who responds only to pain

Subcutaneous emphysema: Air collection under the skin

SVT: Supraventricular Tachycardia (extreme high heart rate which gives feeling of palpitation)

Tachycardia: very high heart rate

TBI: Traumatic Brain Injury (any injury to the brain after head injury-contusion, bleeding etc)

Thrombolysis: an injection that dissolves blood clots

TIA: Transient Ischemic Attack (an episode of stroke-like symptoms for just a few minutes which return to normal quickly)

TIPS: Trans jugular intrahepatic portosystemic shunt (it is a procedure in which stent is placed to reduce excessive pressure in blood vessels of liver)

TMT: Treadmill test (to detect changes in ECG after strenuous physical activity like running)

Toxic shock syndrome: very serious disease caused by bacterial toxins leading to fever, skin rashes and extremely low blood pressure

Tracheostomy: placing a breathing tube through the neck directly into the windpipe

Urosepsis: Severe urinary tract infection which can be life-threatening

UTI: Urinary Tract Infection

Variceal Bleeding: blood in vomiting due to burst veins in the oesophagus (food pipe)

Vasospasm: sudden narrowing of blood vessels causing reduction of blood supply

Vegetative State: Unconscious person who has sleep–wake cycles and may appear awake

VF: Ventricular Fibrillation (extreme high and irregular heart rate which can make patient unresponsive)

VT: Ventricular Tachycardia (extreme high heart rate which can make patient unconscious and unresponsive)

ICU Diary